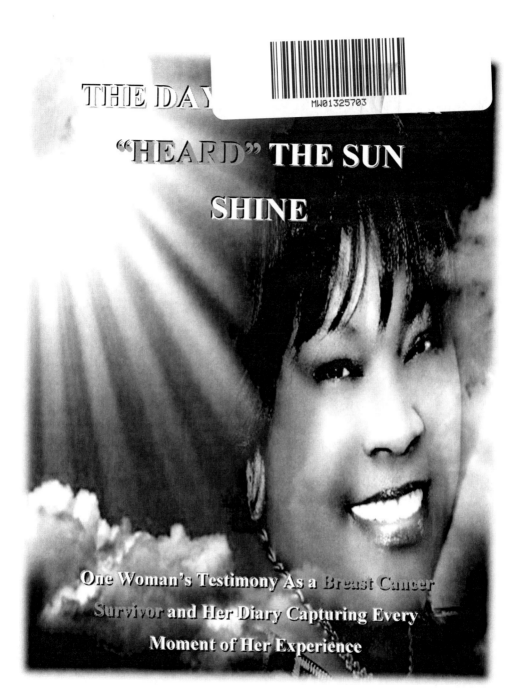

THE DAY I "HEARD" THE SUN SHINE

One Woman's Testimony As a Breast Cancer Survivor and Her Diary Capturing Every Moment of Her Experience

Written By Althea Baldwin

2011 © The Day I No Longer "Heard" The Sun Shine

DIP Publishing House
3500 Riverwood Parkway
Suite 1900
Atlanta, Georgia 30039

Mailing address:
PO BOX 723262
Atlanta, Georgia 31139

© 2011 *Althea Baldwin*
No part of this book may be reproduced, stored in a retrieval system, or transmitted by any means without the written permission of the author.

First published by **DIP Publishing House** 08/01/2011
ISBN: 978-0-9845451-9-3
Library of Congress Control Number: 2011934615

Printed in the United States – Atlanta, Georgia

TABLE OF CONTENTS

FOREWORD

INTRODUCTION

   CHAPTER 1
   THE DAY I NO LONGER
   "HEARD" THE SUN SHINE 17

   CHAPTER 2
   AN UNWELCOMED DISCOVERY 21

   CHAPTER 3
   OFF TO FLORIDA WE GO............................... 26

   CHAPTER 4
   LET THE EXAMINATIONS BEGIN-
   "A DIVINE VISITATION"
   (BRACING FOR THE
   DREADED ANNOUNCEMENT) 30

   CHAPTER 5
   MRI FEARS-
   THE PAIN OF THE RESULTS 50

CHAPTER 6
THANK GOD FOR THE SUPPORT
OF FAMILY AND FRIENDS
"A CELEBRATION OF LOVE" 64

CHAPTER 7
MY FIRST VISIT WITH MY ONCOLOGIST-
A BATTERY OF SCANS AND TESTS 67

CHAPTER 8
HOW SAD TO LEAVE MY JOB
IF ONLY FOR AWHILE 78

CHAPTER 9
THE DELIGHT OF MEETING NEW FRIENDS-I GET
MY FIRST WIG! 82

CHAPTER 10
DISAPPOINTING NEWS-A RESCHEDULE OF MY
FIRST DAY OF CHEMOTHERAPY 86

CHAPTER 11
SECOND BIOPSY-
FOLLOW UP FROM MY PET SCAN
(SUSPICIOUS CELLS) 92

CHAPTER 12
"INDEPENDENCE DAY"-
A CELEBRATION AND TIME OF RELAXATION
WITH MY DAUGHTER (WHAT FUN!).......................... 98

CHAPTER 13
MY SECOND RESCHEDULING TO START FIRST
DAY OF CHEMOTHERAPY.. 110

CHAPTER 14
MY SECOND MRI-
MORE ANXIETY!... 113

CHAPTER 15
A BREAK FROM THE MADNESS-
A HAIR APPOINTMENT AND VISIT TO TV 5
STUDIOS... 118

CHAPTER 16
FIRST OFFICIAL DAY OF CHEMOTHERAPY AND
THE PAINFUL SIDE EFFECTS TO FOLLOW........... 127

CHAPTER 17
OH NO…
THERE GOES MY HAIR!... 136

CHAPTER 18
FIRST SUNDAY
BACK TO CHURCH AFTER 3 MONTHS 141

CHAPTER 19
GOODBYE MRS. SANDERS............................. 146

CHAPTER 20
TREATMENT HALFWAY MARK-AND
"IT'S BRITTANIE'S BIRTHDAY"!....................... 151

CHAPTER 21
LAST DAY OF CHEMOTHERAPY TREATMENT!.. 159

CHAPTER 22
GENERAL ELECTION DAY 2008........................ 163

CHAPTER 23
PREPARING FOR BILATERAL MASTECTOMY
SURGERY-
"JORDYNN HAS A BIRTHDAY"!........................ 171

CHAPTER 24
"THANKSGIVING DAY".................................. 176

CHAPTER 25
CONSULTATION WITH PLASTIC SURGEON BEFORE MASTECTOMY SURGERY 179

CHAPTER 26
MY VISIT BACK TO MY JOB BEFORE SURGERY.. 183

CHAPTER 27
BRITTANIE GRADUATES AND A MEMORABLE DINNER.. 186

CHAPTER 28
MORE PRE-SURGICAL TESTS- "DANA CELEBRATES HER BIRTHDAY"!................. 194

CHAPTER 29
DAY OF SURGERY (BILATERAL MASTECTOMY).. 197

CHAPTER 30
GOING HOME FROM THE HOSPITAL AND THE AFTERMATH 205

CHAPTER 31
CHRISTMAS DAY AND NEW YEAR'S EVE 209

CHAPTER 32
POST BREAST RESTORATION PROCEDURES 214

CHAPTER 33
PAUL AND I CELEBRATE OUR WEDDING ANNIVERSARY-
FOLLOW UP WITH DR. LINDSEY AND DR. HARLAND 218

CHAPTER 34
HERCEPTIN TREATMENTS RESUMED-ECKO CARDIO TESTS 222

CHAPTER 35
CONSULTATION WITH ONCOLOGY RADIOLOGIST TO BEGIN RADIATION
THERAPY TREATMENTS 226

CHAPTER 36
ONCOLOGIST CONFIRMS NEED FOR RADIATION TREATMENT-DISAPPOINTING NEWS 230

CHAPTER 37
BREAST RESTORATION
 PROCEDURES RESUMED 235

CHAPTER 38
**MOTHER BERNICE MURPHY-
WHAT A VISIT!** 238

CHAPTER 39
BREAST IMPLANT SURGERY 245

CHAPTER 40
**PREPARATION FOR
RADIATION TREATMENT** 247

CHAPTER 41
**GEORGIA CANCER CENTER ORDERS
ANOTHER CT SCAN** 252

CHAPTER 42
**LAST DAY OF RADIATION TREATMENT AND THE
END OF HERCEPTIN TREATMENT** 254

CHAPTER 43
**MY FIRST SPEAKING ENGAGEMENT AS BREAST
CANCER SURVIVOR** 257

CHAPTER 44
**MY PORT IS SURGICALLY REMOVED FROM MY
CHEST-
A "CLEAN BILL OF HEALTH"!** 260

CHAPTER 45
SO WHERE DO I GO FROM HERE
AND WHAT HAVE I LEARNED 263

ACKNOWLEDGEMENTS

SPECIAL DEDICATION
TO MY LOVING HUSBAND & CHILDREN 276

RESOURCES
(ORGANIZATIONS THAT HELP CANCER PATIENTS) 280

ABOUT THE AUTHOR 283

FOREWORD

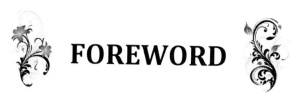

This book was written from the heart. If you are a woman who is struggling with what to expect as it relates to breast cancer, or if you know other women who are struggling this is the BOOK to READ. Althea Baldwin took the time to share her personal story in a detailed "unique" way. She not only shared her story she shared her family as well. I salute Mrs. Baldwin for having the resilience and faith to conquer breast cancer. I also commend her for the compassion she has for others as she has become a beacon of hope to those who need comfort in this area.

-Donna Warfield Fareed
Amazon Best Selling Author
"Whatever Floats Your Boat"

INTRODUCTION

When I was diagnosed with breast cancer in June 2008, I'd never known how one's life could be suddenly turned upside down. We all have goals and aspirations that we desire to achieve, never anticipating obstacles that would deem those goals unachievable. My life literally stalled, and hurled itself into a black hole of uncertainty. Living this healthy life, I never imagined that I would be diagnosed with such a dreadful disease. Against all odds, we set our goals naturally and spiritually and we fight with everything within us to achieve them. I knew I had a challenge ahead of me that required strong faith in God. If not for my faith and knowing that God completely controls our lives as He wills, I would not have made it through this journey. A journey it was, and I now live each day of my life telling my story to women everywhere who desire to have their faith strengthened.

One should live a life enriched with meaning, purpose, and substance. One may feel they are living all they know to live and doing all they know to do to make their lives complete. But everyone experiences moments of despair when we ask ourselves…"am I living my life the way that God expects me to? Many questions flood our minds…"am I being that example that others can look upon and be proud"? "What can I do in my life that would better serve others?" I felt I had come to that point in my life before my illness. Whether one agrees with the thought or not, I believe the Lord causes life changing events in our lives that allow us to reflect upon the quality of our lives and our purpose. My diagnosis was the catalyst that helped me realize what was most important in my life. I considered myself to be a true Christian, yet I lacked the evidence and level of power of God in my life I desired. I felt my spirit spiraling downward in an abyss. I needed something, someone in my life to strengthen my spiritual man. The Lord is Omnipotent and knows our every need. He is mindful of our physical and spiritual state in life. He knows how to bring us back to a life in him that is according to his Will. He will fill every void we experience and restore a fulfilled life. I could only cry to the Lord in my despair, as spoken in Psalms 61:2 "From the end of the earth will I cry unto thee, when my heart is overwhelmed: lead me to the rock that is higher than I". I knew I needed help beyond my own strength. Little did I know that my moment of change would be met with a life changing health diagnosis that literally saved my life! I could not see that when I was ill, but the journey I traveled throughout this time in my life proved phenomenally miraculous. I had no idea how I would get through this test, but I knew I had to.

    I wanted to be that example that the Word of God speaks of in Romans 12:3... "For I say, through the grace given unto me, to every man that is among you, not to think of himself more highly than he ought to think; but to think soberly, according as God has dealt to every man the *measure of faith*". I have always wanted my "measure of faith" to compliment the test I was given. Without faith...it is truly impossible to please God. I learned how to clearly discern the voice of the Lord through this suffering. His voice is all we have to guide us through trials of peril. "Cancer" can be a dark tunnel to travel and certainly intimidating, but I can now say that I'm grateful to have had this experience. I would love to share my journey with all who would take this ride with me. I pray that it will bless you as it has me. I also offer you hope in the midst of tragedy.

When the Lord spoke to me and asked me to document my journey, my body was so riddled with pain that I didn't know how I could physically keep my head up, not to mention write the details of my experience. I wrote of my experiences just as I was spiritually led to do it through a diary. My experiences will be relived from the first day of my learning of my diagnosis, through every examination, test, procedure, surgery, various treatments, reconstruction, and recovery. As difficult as it was journaling this diary of events, I found it therapeutic to do it. You will note that I wrote each experience on the exact day of the event and my emotions reflect the mental state I was in during that moment. My emotions were extreme from one end of the spectrum to the other. Nevertheless, the need to share what the Lord was doing for me through each experience was essential in telling my story. It is my desire that this book will serve as a reference guide to breast cancer patients in what to expect in the next step of their experience. If I can help relieve the fear, I will have assisted in helping another find comfort in this journey. I pray my story touches your life and causes your faith to soar into the heart of God!

As a final note, names and facilities have been changed to protect the privacy of individuals involved.

CHAPTER 1
THE DAY I NO LONGER "HEARD" THE SUN SHINE

There will be a day that comes along in everyone's life, when life as you've known it before, completely changes and starts anew. Sometimes that life-changing experience comes through great pain and suffering, with unknown joy to follow. It is a great day when one can go outside and see the sun shine, feel its warmth on their skin and see its glowing rays illuminate the earth. There is even a sense of hearing the sun shining with all its might, when one is lounging on a sunlit patio, asleep or resting on a sunny beach taking in its rays. If you listen closely, you can actually **hear** the sun saying… "relax… enjoy…let me wrap you in my warm arms!" But there is another day when your very soul diminishes in mid air...when that air seemingly takes you worlds below the surface of the earth. No longer do you feel the sun's rays, or see its aluminous glow; neither can you feel the warmth on your skin. You no longer **hear** those sounds of brightness or shouts of gleam that only the sun can project. It's like you're in a dark world all alone listening to the only voice(s) that speaks...telling you news of tragic proportion. That news can come in the form of your health, finances, relationship, or spirituality. My tragic news came when I heard the words "you have cancer". Hearing these words caused all of my senses to completely shut down. I could not see, hear, or speak. Thus, I experienced a sensation of the inability to see or *hear* the sun in my life. Nevertheless, there is no sound from the sun to tell us that everything will be alright. We then listen to the voice of the Lord to hear comfort, peace, love, and assurance...*He is the source of our sun.* We look to the Lord to warm us, to glow through us as His servants...*He is the source of our sun.* We look to the Lord for those rays that reflect our own lives as His...*He is the source of our sun.* When we listen to His voice... "like a trumpet crying out in the wilderness"...*He is the most powerful* *source of our sun.* A sheep knows His Father's voice and a stranger it will not listen to or follow (St. John 10:27). The good Shepherd surrounds us with His love and comforts us with protection we've never known. It is my desire, that "the day you no longer hear your sun shine or hear its voice…you will listen to the voice of the Lord". He is even nearer to you than the sun. He is crying out to you with a loud voice, or maybe in a whisper that "He's never left you". He's never relinquished His stand on your behalf, He will always be there whenever you need him. He's a God that begat the sun to shine, glow, touch us, and allows us to hear its every call. Just listen!

(SYNOPSIS OF JOURNAL)

The following is a detailed account of my life May 12, 2008 to the present. It was this day, unknowing to me, that would serve as the turning point in my life and all that I knew and held dear was viewed through a totally different lens. No one knows the day or the hour that the Lord will reappear or return to this earth…but one thing we do know is that our lives are in His HOLY hands and what He chooses to do with it is entirely His divine desire and WILL. He did it with my life…and I love him for every step of my journey. Please follow along with me on this sometimes surprisingly and uncertain walk…

CHAPTER 2
AN UNWELCOMED DISCOVERY

Monday, May 12, 2008- On this day after feeling a rather HUGE lump in my breast, I decided to visit my Gynecologist Dr. Donald Yancey, who has been my Gynecologist now for nearly 36 years. I felt this lump for the first time in April 2008. I clearly remember my visit with Dr. Yancey on this date, because it was on this date that my company, ADOLESCENT PREGNANCY PREVENTION OF GEORGIA (APPG) celebrated our annual Premiere event. A Premiere is APPG's annual celebration and fund raiser featured with a movie or various accomplishments on screen related to pregnancy prevention. Dr. Yancey examined my breasts and realized that there was a noticeable mass in my left breast that needed further examination via mammogram. I normally have my annual mammograms at the Cytec Radiology Center. I had my mammogram at this facility every year after I turned 50. I had my very first mammogram when I was 37. I left Dr. Yancey's office with nervous anticipation of having this mammogram done, and uncertain what this large lump would mean. Whatever my emotions, I went ahead and attended my company's Annual Premiere with a quiet prayer in my spirit, not saying anything to ANYONE...not even my husband, Paul. He never even knew I made the appointment with Dr. Yancey or with Cytec Radiology.

I wanted to vacation in Deltona, Florida the week of May 19th 2008 to go visit my parents. After all, I had planned twice to go see them and both visits were cancelled due to circumstances beyond my control. With such an overprotective husband, I knew if he knew my health situation, he would not allow me to go see my parents. He loved my parents and would have gone in a heartbeat, but for Paul, my health came first, and understandably so. Making this visit to see them meant the world to me! So I said nothing to him about my health...nothing at all.

Wednesday, May 14, 2008-I visited Cytec Radiology for my mammogram. The month of May would have served as my annual mammogram month anyway, since I'd just had my previous one, May 2007. After visiting the Radiology Center, they processed my normal mammogram, but then decided that I needed to go on into the next room for further tests which consisted of an ultrasound. I still told my husband... nothing.

Friday, May 16, 2008- Dr. Yancey reviewed my x-rays from Cytec Radiology and called me. He informed me that there was something *suspicious* seen during my ultrasound and mammogram. Reports never tell you exactly what they see; only that something *suspicious* was found. By this time, I was feeling quite anxious, because the week of May 19th meant "*VACATION*" for me... and seeing my parents. Oh how I had waited to see them... like a little girl! Dr. Yancey referred me to a Breast Specialist at the Breast Cancer Care Center. I then told Dr. Yancey that I would certainly follow up with the Breast Care Center he'd recommended, but I asked him if it was alright if I go on vacation first. I promised him I would see the Specialist as soon as I was back in town. He agreed, but firmly advised that I keep this appointment. I agreed. He asked me to go by the Radiology Center to pick up my films and take them in hand to the Breast Cancer Care Center...and report to Dr. Nancy Harland. Still... I told Paul nothing.

Week of May 19th, 2008-After pondering over and over in my mind, should I go see my parents or should I stay and go to this appointment that Dr. Yancey insisted I keep my appointment with the Breast Cancer Center...I said a prayer and decided to leave for Florida on Friday, May 23rd. All this time I was deciding whether I should go visit my parents or stay home. I still had not whispered a word of my x-ray findings to Paul. Still hoping and praying Paul would insist that I not go on my vacation due to the discovery on my mammogram and ultrasound...I waited until mid week to tell him what was found. I finally told Paul the truth about the findings on my screenings. He was stunned to say the least and deeply concerned about my health. He did not want me to go to Florida alone with my two grandchildren. He insisted that he go with me. I was so thrilled to hear him say that, it brought me to tears. I wanted him to go with me to see my parents all along, and now I got my wish! Besides, I really needed him with me during this uncertain and frightening time in my life.

CHAPTER 3
OFF TO FLORIDA WE GO

Friday, May 23, 2008-My daughter Dana, and her friend Derron, decided to drive their vehicle to Florida along with her daughter Amaya, my granddaughter. Their whole purpose of going to Florida was to take Amaya to Disney World...mine was to see my parents, vacation, and relax! Paul decided to drive our car. Previously, I was going to drive alone with our two granddaughters. I must have been out of my mind, thinking I could drive alone with a 1 and a 4 year old. I wanted desperately to go! Paul watched me like a hawk and made sure I did no heavy lifting, exhaustive work, or over exertion. That's pretty difficult not to do, especially going to visit my parents (smile). Our original plan was for me to drive alone with my grandbabies, and then Paul would come down toward the end of my trip to pick me and the grandbabies up, and then drive us back home to Atlanta. But when he heard of my diagnosis, *all systems were go* for him to drive down with me.

We prayed and ventured off on this vacation with one thought in mind, we would go to Florida, have a really wonderful time, relax, and above all, tell my parents not one word about my health discovery. We had a real ball! I loved how my granddaughter, Amaya's eyes lit up after visiting Disney with her Mom and Dad. Every one of her Disney dreams came true! That made the whole entire trip worthwhile. It was nice to watch my granddaughter, Jordynn bring so much joy to my parents' eyes while she ran around the house, laughing and playing. That made the trip one of the best I've had. It was so delightful!

My Mom and Dad drove us to a park near their home. They sat outside with Paul and I, and enjoyed watching the grandbabies run, play, and tire themselves out having so much fun. My Mom, who has limited mobility with walking without the use of a wheelchair, walker, or cane, walked slowly with her walker and acted like a kid herself. It was all so breathtaking for me. It was refreshing to watch our parents enjoying themselves with the grandchildren. For a time, I was able to become pleasantly distracted. In the back of my mind, I never stopped thinking about my health issue I had to face when I got back home to Atlanta.

Monday, May 26, 2008-My dad, who I've never considered a cooking or grilling man, stayed on the grill all morning and prepared us the best Memorial Day feast. We enjoyed barbecue ribs, chicken, hotdogs, and hamburgers. We feasted the entire week on all these succulent meats. He scorched a few ribs and chicken, but it didn't matter, every bite was filled with love! (smile)

Saturday, May 31, 2008-With tears in our eyes, and two little tired sleepy grandbabies that woke up too early in the morning from their vacation, we prepared to leave my parents and go back home to Atlanta to face the inevitable. Of course the trip back home with an 18 month old and 4 year old in the car for a 6 hour drive would not be complete without a portable DVD player in the back seats. We purchased dual screens for each of them to view. Featured for their viewing pleasure were their favorite Disney princesses and characters. It really did the trick for the long ride back.

They sang along with the DVDS and were quite occupied. I was so glad... I needed to relax my mind...just a little.

CHAPTER 4
LET THE EXAMINATIONS BEGIN-
"A DIVINE VISITATION"

(BRACING FOR THE DREADED ANNOUNCEMENT)

Monday, June 2, 2008- I went to a routine follow up appointment with my PCP, Dr. Harold Dressler. This was simply to have him go over lab results, unrelated to my breast tests. I consider Dr. Dressler not only my doctor, but also a spiritual friend. We can never leave his office without sharing about the Lord. He surprisingly had already obtained the written report from my mammogram and ultrasound tests taken at Cytec Radiology. For the first time, I had a chance to read the results in detail. I saw the measurement of my lump in my breast and learned of other tumors that were found as well. There were tumors found in both breasts, but mainly in the left breast. On a scale called the **ACR BI-RADS Mammographic codes scale** of 1-6, the report stated that the lump in the left breast was rated as a category 5, which is malignant. The report further read that an irregular nodule measured approximately 2.3 cm in greatest dimension. The nodule was solid. Another solid nodule measured 1.0 cm in greatest dimension. Adjacent to this, a smaller sub centimeter cyst was noted. Biopsy was highly recommended. My heart dropped, but yet I prayed. Dr. Dressler informed me of the nature of my tumor rating and assured me that we would pray and believe God for a miracle that it would not be anymore serious than expected. I left his office that day, confident that our prayers would sustain me for what I was getting ready to experience.

Monday, June 2, 2008- After leaving Dr. Dressler's office I stopped by Cytec Radiology and picked up my x-ray results as I was instructed to by Dr. Yancey.

Tuesday, June 3, 2008- I returned to work from my vacation. I told only my Supervisor, Cindy Taylor and our HR Director, Alyssa Walters of my news. I quietly went to work and performed my duties while mentally numb. I could not concentrate on any of my work as I should.

Monday, June 9, 2008-This day will be a day that I will never forget. It was on this date that I had my appointment with the Breast Cancer Care Center with Dr. Nancy Harland. Dr. Harland was a renowned breast Surgeon. I went to the office with x-ray results in hand to take to Dr. Harland, as instructed by Dr. Yancey. I must say that this day was pretty routine…or so I thought. I went in and registered at the reception desk feeling that same confidence that I felt when I left Dr. Dressler's office. The Breast Cancer office mailed at least 5-6 pages of very important paperwork that I had to complete before being seen by the doctor. In these pre-registered papers, you are warned that your first visit may take at least 3-4 hours. So I was prepared for the long wait. I completed additional paper work, submitted my insurance information and then waited for further instructions. I became anxious because the clerk told me that they had not received my referral from Dr. Yancey's office. I wondered what could have happened to it. I'd preregistered with Dr. Yancey's office for this appointment. Certainly they processed my information. The clerk allowed me to proceed to the next waiting area while they pursued my referral information.

I was then instructed to change into the gown provided. I was escorted into the next room where women sat by the dozens awaiting to have a mammogram or ultrasound done or simply wait for the final step...to see the Surgeon. The office is a pretty remarkable place, and is very professionally operated. Women are systematically directed to areas of the office based on your needs. I was impressed that all Surgeons on staff were female. There were about 4 or 5 Doctors on staff. Pretty amazing team!

I was escorted to the small room where another ultrasound was taken of my left breast. I had taken this test many times in the past, but for the first time ever, the technician asked me to speak...to simply say a few words. I found that rather strange. I'd never been asked to speak before. Of course, in my curiosity, I asked the young lady what was the purpose of asking me to speak? She replied that an ultrasound is mechanically guided by sound. By speaking and hearing the patient's voice, it targets certain organs, muscles and vessels to locate them on screen. I was pretty fascinated!

I must caution you before reading the following experience. I am sharing it from a **spiritual point of view. I pray that I can relay my experience to you in the same sense that I experienced it, and that it will be a blessing to you. **

The technician walks out of the room to develop the x-ray film and have the Radiologist review them. I lay there on the table in pretty wonderful spirits. Then all of a sudden, it seemed as though my body, mind, and spirit became overwhelmingly overtaken by a spirit of "Praise and Worship". It suddenly appeared that the Lord took control of my mind and it was no longer mine. It was an incredible moment to behold! I began to hear the song in my spirit…"LIKE NEVER BEFORE" by Minister William Murphy. This is a remarkably popular worship and praise song. Anyone in the presence of this song is tremendously blessed. That song played over and over in my mind and ministered to me like I've never heard it minister before. The Lord began to minister through the words of this song to me… "A like never before Praise…A like never before Word, A like never before Passion, A like never before Cry, A like never before Release." I've never experienced such a rippling sensation in my heart and spirit. It's like the Lord was preparing me for something to come…but what was it? In all my faith in the Lord, I could not see that he was preparing me for such a life changing moment. The song kept ministering to me. The words of the song went on to say "Lord, I want more of you…more of your power, more of your glory, more of you Lord!" To hunger for more of the Lord's spirit like you've never hungered for him before is such an overpowering experience. This hunger causes your desires to no longer be your own. You completely submit your life to God's Will. That's what the Lord was saying to me through this song. How amazing. The song finally concluded that "I want more of you Lord, not like the last time". This hunger created a yearning and desire in me I'd never had before. What an extraordinary experience! I became overcome with emotion.

The Lord then preached the most powerful sermon through me. I was audibly saying the words that the Lord was speaking to my spirit. I cried with uncontrollable tears. He began to tell me how I was getting ready to go to a level in Him that I'd never experienced before. He told me "that His Words will no longer mean the same to me as before". "The songs I hear of Him will not be the same songs I knew before, but will be songs that will break yokes not only in my life but the lives of others." He said "when you minister to others, chains will break and closed ears will be open like I've never seen before." Then suddenly the entire small room where I lay began to separate itself from its foundation…and I began to float in air. I felt so light and lifted. The tears would not stop flowing. It seemed that nothing was any longer in my hands, but all released to Him. I've never in my life had this kind of experience. I have had awesome moments with the Lord in my life…but this was very DIFFERENT, and so AMAZING. I loved every minute of it. The Lord saturated me with his presence, his warmth, and his love. I cannot even explain this moment!

As my spiritual experience continued…I then remembered one of the last Bible Study services that I attended at my church. My Pastor's wife, Evangelist Carolyn Vinson asked if anyone wanted to come up for prayer at the end of services. I alone walked up. I felt such a desire in my heart to go up to the altar and surround myself with the corporate prayers of the Saints. I have always embraced the power of corporate prayer. There is awesome strength in allowing God's people to pray for and with you. Evangelist Vinson prayed a powerfully anointed prayer. I felt engulfed in God's presence. Others began to come up to the Altar for prayer. I could feel their cries and hear their weeping along with my own. I then heard Evangelist Vinson say these profound words…she said "many of you have come up and are asking for a closer walk with the Lord and now He has given you this great opportunity! Allow him to use you, and walk in this new calling and new elevation in Him." I am actually paraphrasing what Evangelist Vinson said, but it was all the voice of the Lord speaking, and as close to what the Lord said through her as I can recall. It was an evening Bible Study, and prayer that I'll never forget!

****

The ultrasound technician comes back into the room, but my sermon is now over. As quickly as I was thrust into my "*out of body*" experience... the Lord has placed me back on solid ground...lying there on that table. It was a moment exemplifying a dream. The technician was so pleasant. It appeared that she took a moment to look at me, as though she even noticed something different about me. It was such a memorable experience!

After my ultrasound, I was then escorted to the next waiting area. This room sat outside the door of the Surgeon's office. In my case, I patiently awaited Dr. Harland's nurse to call my name. While I was waiting, I called Dr. Yancey's office to ask them to PLEASE fax over my referral to the BREAST CANCER CENTER office. I was concerned that if the BREAST CANCER CENTER office did not receive Dr. Yancey's office paperwork, I would have to pay "out of pocket" expenses, of which I wasn't prepared to pay.

Dr. Yancey's office assured me that they faxed my referral over when I requested it days prior, but due to the large volume of patients, at the BREAST CANCER CENTER office, the fax phone line was constantly busy. Finally, I found out during my wait to go into Dr. Harland's office, they had resolved the fax problem and submitted it to the BREAST CANCER CENTER office. I breathed a sigh of relief! I am feeling so confident and relaxed at this point.

I was still emotionally charged from the spiritual experience I had in the ultrasound room. What a moment! But what did it all mean? I began to watch intense expressions on many of the women's faces. I really did not know what they'd experienced, or were preparing to experience. Their experiences ranged from follow up checkups after major surgeries, follow up visits for test results, as well as follow up for maintenance procedures after cancer treatments. Some women wore caps, scarves, and head coverings after the loss of their hair due to cancer. I was unable to relate to many of these women's plights with cancer. I could not comprehend what they'd gone through, nor did I feel I needed to. I couldn't have been more wrong. Nevertheless, I sat and smiled at many of the women without a friendly response in return. I was so removed from the real essence of one's visit to this office...totally clueless.

After waiting nearly an hour, they called my name. I went back to Dr. Harland's office being guided by her nurse. I am singing a song, and nonchalantly strolling my way back to her office. In my mind, I am feeling this is a routine examination. I never expected anything extraordinary would be found. Even after seeing my reports that revealed that my tumor discovery was based on a category 5 on a scale from 1-6, I never expected anything but the best news. I am a praying 'Woman and a Woman of Great Faith'. I knew the Lord would shield me and not give me any bad news....well... so I thought!
Dr. Harland immediately came into the room to see me. I thought she was the most charming doctor with the kind of spunk that matched my mood for that entire day. I imagined what bad news she could give me, with a smile and vibrant spirit such as hers! She escorted me into the next room where she could get better lighting from her x-ray screen viewer. She

reviewed my x-rays with intense concern. She spoke emphatically yet assuredly. She showed me the film on screen and pointed to exactly where the tumors were in my breast. What she said next made my heart drop. She said, not only are there tumors in your breast but also in your lymph nodes. I was not processing or comprehending anything she was explaining to me. Then she shared the words with me that *rendered my body limp and detached.* She said, "Mrs. Baldwin, you have CANCER"! She said that there are surgeries that can remove lumps or if necessary remove the breast. She gave me a minute to catch my breath… and she held my hand. She then said with a comfortable smile on her face… "there is reconstructive surgery that can be done to repair and replace breasts and give women a look and reassurance that will help them reclaim their lives." She further said, "I want to immediately start you on chemotherapy, and after 3 treatments, I want you to come back to me and we will see if the cells are responding before we perform surgery". I'm taking all this in…but AM I? She held my hand while I cried…well, I think I did…I'm not sure what I was doing. My head was totally detached from my body, and my mind was sitting over in the corner of the room staring into space. I cannot explain to you what I was feeling...I just felt my entire body become detached. She asked if I wanted to call my husband. She left the room to give me privacy to talk. What do I say to him? How do I tell him I have cancer? I could not even get THAT word out! For an instant, the Lord reminded me of the experience I'd just previously had in the ultrasound room. It all began to make sense. He was preparing me for this moment...Oh my God...what a moment!

Now I'm sitting in the office alone...and I'm trying to dial Paul. Before I could even dial, I have this war going on in my mind saying... "Lord, this can't be you...you said in your word that by your stripes I am healed!" You even said "that if we have the faith the size of a mustard seed...we could move mountains!" I'm sitting in this room with all these scriptures going over and over in my mind...and saying how could this be happening? God, where are you? I don't remember saying *why me*...I just remember asking...WHY? I continue with this battle going on in my mind.

Of all days of keeping my cell phone charged at ALL times; my phone is now beeping and going dead. OH MY GOD! I had to call Paul, I had to say something to someone, but WHAT? I get a call through to Paul. I told him the news. I remember him saying that he wished he was with me. I went alone, because I honestly didn't expect anything more than a routine examination. I could hear the hurt and disappointment in his voice. I finish the call with Paul and ask him please don't say anything to the girls...my daughters, Dana and Brittanie.

Dr. Harland comes back into the room, gives me tissue and talks to me more in her warm and comforting voice. She then says that she wants to go ahead and prepare me for a biopsy immediately. My mind is still detached, and I didn't even have time to think of *biopsy*...is that going to hurt...will it be uncomfortable? I'm just floating on air and realized that they'd taken me to another room and had me laid out on a table. I remember a very sweet nurse technician came in to assist Dr. Harland. In the midst of my astonishment over the news I'd just received, and the procedure they were getting ready to perform on me, I told the technician how her smile made me feel comfortable as she proceeded to prepare for the procedure. She was a technician who administered the ultrasound or whatever the equipment was that guided Dr. Harland's needle for the biopsy. The technician kept insisting on giving me Kleenex tissue. By now, the tears were really flowing! She was so consoling.

The technician then let me hear the sound that I would hear with the device Dr. Harland would use to shoot the area of the breast and extract tissue for biopsy review. It was the sound similar to a staple gun. Dr. Harland came in to start the procedure. She explained every step of the procedure and told me everything she was doing. She then numbed my breast with a local anesthesia and began the procedure. I remember hearing that staple gun sound at least 6-7 times. All I remember thinking while laying on that table was, please just hurry up with what you have to do and let me go home…I just wanted to get out of there! I could not believe all this was happening to me. It seemed like it was happening to someone else. After the procedure was complete, Dr. Harland told me that she would immediately send my sample tissue to the Pathology department at Northwest Hospital for them to biopsy. She assured me that they were the best and she would have the results in a couple of days. I just remembered saying to myself, I want to leave! The tears just flowed.

Dr. Harland escorted me to the scheduling office to meet Belinda. She told me she was an awesome girl and she'd been a part of this staff for 8 years. Belinda also assured me that I was in the best hands with Dr. Harland. I'd already felt comfortable with Dr. Harland. I just WANTED TO GO HOME! Belinda set up my next appointment with the office. I had a total mental collapse and could not remember my next scheduled appointment. I couldn't comprehend ANYTHING. I JUST WANTED TO GO HOME! I asked Dr. Harland if I could go back to work. She said only if I had to; but to go home shortly after that and get some rest. She warned me that the local anesthesia from the biopsy procedure would wear off within a couple of hours. I JUST WANTED TO GO HOME…but decided to go back to work. I really needed to occupy my mind with work, and suddenly I DIDN'T WANT TO GO HOME!

I went on to work, and talked with Paul all the way to my job. I remember calling Tina, my friend and co-worker and telling her my news. Her heart dropped and she became so quiet...just lost for words. Tina always had a word of encouragement when we talked, but this time she could only say, "we will talk when you get into the office." I arrived at work, at approximately 2:00 in the afternoon. I sat in my car for awhile in the parking lot and talked to Dana, my daughter, and cried even more. I told her the news. She assured me... "Mommy we will get through this with faith and prayer." I have a praying family and that was reassuring. Her voice was so soothing!

I finally got out of my car and went into the office. Just as I got off the elevator and began to step into my office, my daughter Brittanie called. She was in her last semester before graduating college. She was studying Broadcast Journalism. She was interning with TV 5 News and had just left out of their daily meeting. In these meetings she received instructions on news stories that she would go on along with reporters she would shadow. Her voice is all bubbly...she's always excited when going out. She asked how my visit at the Doctor's office went. Well of course I don't want her to know any of my news yet. I wanted to keep her focused on her news report for the day. So I quietly told her they were still awaiting results and I would follow up with her later. All of this time I'm dying inside from the news I'd just learned. I hated lying to her, but I knew I couldn't tell her the truth at this time. She excitedly told me about her very first news story with TV 5 News that she was about to cover and hurriedly got off the phone. I stayed outside my office doors next to the elevator and cried uncontrollably. I decided then to tell Brittanie after she came home from her internship after 12:00 midnight.

I immediately stopped by my HR Director Alyssa's office. I told her my news. She encouraged me as only she could...with every scripture of assurance, to stand on my faith and trust God to get me through this. I walked to my desk as though I was in a daze and began to work. As the afternoon went on, I began to feel stinging in my breast. The feeling was coming back from my procedure, I then decided to go on home. I remember working until nearly 6:30 that evening. I couldn't believe that I actually stayed and worked that long…everyone in the office had left and gone home…and I never even realized it!

Wednesday, June 11, 2008- I received a call from Dr. Harland with my biopsy test results from Pathology. She confirmed what she'd already told me June 9th from the x-rays and ultrasound that the results were malignant tumors. She then told me that she had to order an MRI exam. I didn't know the extent of an MRI exam, but I knew I was very claustrophobic. After going online and researching the procedure, I knew I wouldn't last 1 minute in that environment. No way, No how! I am a praying woman, but God himself wasn't taking me in that machine…uh uh! (smile).
Dr. Harland then promised she'd call me back with contacts to see a good Oncologist near my area of town in South Fulton. I was blessed to be referred by her to the Georgia Cancer Center office

in Fayetteville, under the care of Dr. Iyam Sharian. He along with his personal nurse, Molly, had become my lifeline to this dreaded disease. They have made my perception less frightening and more comforting. I couldn't thank them more.

CHAPTER 5

MRI FEARS—

THE PAIN OF THE

RESULTS

Friday, June 13, 2008- Guess what this day is...I'm scheduled for my very first MRI at the BREAST CANCER CENTER office. This would be the first day of one of the most frightening experiences I can say that I've experienced up to this point in my life. I told you about my claustrophobia. Enclosed small places will serve as my ultimate death. I always said if our country ever went to war on our soil, and the only source of escape or shelter was to enter a tunnel below or above ground where darkness capsules me...I will kiss each one of my family members goodbye and tell them that I'd meet them on the other side ...heaven. (smile) There's no way I would survive this kind of experience.

Little did I know that I could have been medicated to undergo this procedure but I'm sure Dr. Harland as well as the MRI technicians wanted to see how I'd do alone without the medication. A very nice technician nurse was so accommodating in preparing me for the procedure. She had me store all personal effects under the table of the bed where I was being prepped for the procedure. She verified all my medical information on my questionnaire to make sure I didn't have metal plates in my head, nose, ears or any other strange areas of my body! (smile) I then remembered and reminded her of a horrible car accident that I was involved in with my girls back in 1990. I told her I suffered serious head injury. My husband and family had always teased me that I had a metal plate in my head that would cause the metal detectors at the airport to always go off! (smile) Well, being in the mental state that I was in during that head injury surgery and the aftermath of my life…I didn't know or remember if a metal plate was inserted or not. I just went ahead on the premise that I really might have something in my head that would cause this machine to malfunction on me. If I did have a metal plate in my head, I thought, that would have been good news that could possibly cancel my visit...right? WRONG!

After another technician inserted an Intravenous (**IV**) in my arm to inject dye, they decided to go ahead and escort me into the MRI room. I was in lofty spirits until I got into the actual room that housed the dreaded MRI "*contraption*"! (smile) I could immediately feel myself shutting down. To see this little space capsule that was supposed to house my "*overweightness*" (smile), I knew it was going to be an interesting ride! I can't imagine the bravery the astronauts possess in climbing into one of these things... how extraordinary... what courage!

Well, they get me to lie on this table that slides into this space-like capsule, but first there are a lot of adjustments to be made. First of all, you're lying face down on your stomach, then your two breasts are hanging through these two holes that serve to hold them in place. I'm pretty large breasted, so it took some pulling and tugging to get me positioned. Once the stomach is flat on the table, the breasts are resting comfortably in these two huge holes then your face is placed in a massage table type mask that gives airway to your mouth and nose. So it sounds safe...right? Well, until I had to then stretch my arms straight out over my head holding onto two bars to hold me in place. Sounds like a pretty *comfy* position right? WRONG! I'm all in place and ready to slide into this little capsule right? Well, each time I lay my face down in this mask I keep raising up trying to breathe...just to catch my breath a little. Well each time I did that, the technicians tell me that I have to lie still and NOT MOVE, or I will totally distort the entire test. They assured me that there is air flowing up to my face that will cause me to breathe normally. Well, I'm trying with everything in me to make this work...after all I know how important this test is for me to proceed to the next step in my cancer cure. But Lord knows, I actually could not breathe! I began to hyperventilate and experience a panic attack unlike anything I've ever experienced in my entire life! I knew, and they knew I couldn't go through with it. So they take me off the table before they even slid me into this small capsule... and by the way, this was what is called a *closed MRI* as opposed to an *open MRI* which most ladies advised me to try.

Unfortunately for me, the BREAST CANCER CENTER office only has closed MRI's (smile). I am crying crocodile tears and I am somewhat embarrassed by my actions.

Once I was unable to proceed with the procedure, the original technician that saw me came in and immediately asked the other technicians to take me out of the machine. They took me off the table and escorted me into a sitting area right outside the MRI screening room. She talked to me so calmly and said that I might need to have meds given to me to undergo the procedure. But I'd have to come back for a rescheduled appointment. At that point, I really didn't care, I just knew that I couldn't go back through that again in my present mental state. The feeling of not being able to catch my next breath made me feel that I would experience a heart attack! The technician began to share God's Word with me via scriptures that promised peace and comfort. She told me "that the Lord would not bring me to this point to leave me." I knew her words were true and confirmation in my spirit of what I know of God's Word. I responded to her with a smile and she proceeded to get instructions from the doctors on the furtherance of my procedure. One of the other technicians began to comfort me as well and tell me that many women have this very same experience...don't feel bad. I appreciated her encouragement, but I still felt bad because I felt that I'd imposed on their time and schedule, not to mention that this would delay my progress.

My obvious fears along with my admitting that I'd probably had a metal plate in my head gave the technician and Doctors concern to have me leave the MRI office immediately and go next door to an x-ray facility to schedule an x-ray of my head. They wanted to be assured I had no metal plate in my head. This was very important before they could proceed to reschedule an appointment for another MRI. Paul and I left very disappointed that we had to go to another Specialist to get tests done that would further prolong my procedure. We found the x-ray office a couple of streets over from the BREAST CANCER CENTER's office. We went into Bearingway Radiation Clinic and had the x-rays done pretty quickly, got our film printout and immediately dropped them back off at the BREAST CANCER CENTER office. Paul parked the car in front of the BREAST CANCER CENTER office and ran the x-ray film upstairs to them. He had been so supportive of me through every step of my process and knew how to expedite a whole lot of time...he was always the best. He too knew that time was of the essence!

Wednesday, June 18, 2008- Well, this is my second try for the MRI procedure. However, this time Dr. Harland has called in medication for me to take to calm my nerves so that I can go through with it. I'm asked to take the medication ½ hour before the procedure. I check into the Breast Cancer Center office at 10:30 a.m. for an 11:00 a.m. appointment. I went ahead and took my medication at 10:20, as soon as I checked in. I wanted to make sure I was properly medicated and not remember anything...if possible! (smile)

The same young lady, who was my original technician from my first visit, came out to greet me and to escort me back for the procedure. She teased me and asked if I was ready this time?! I assured her I was.

She verified that I had taken my medication to calm my nerves...then jokingly remarked that I'll be just fine this time! (smile)   We went through the same procedures as before and I was given my IV for dye injection and placed properly on the table for the procedure.

Patients are allowed to bring relaxing music that is played through headphones. I brought my Women's Choir CD to play during the procedure. This was the most peaceful and relaxing worship CD imaginable. The CD had a beautiful worship song on it written by Evangelist Vinson.   She shared her testimony of her own bout with breast cancer. It was all very calming. I also remembered, another sister from my church, Sis. Leslie Hill. She'd also overcome a serious bout of lung cancer and she knew my fear of the MRI. She sent a most powerful e-mail to me that I read the morning before I left home for the procedure. In the e-mail it told a story of an old Indian tale. In order for an Indian lad to show that he was a real man, his dad would take him out in the middle of the forest in the dark of night surrounded by fierce wolves, and animals of every kind. The young boy would be blind folded and left on a stump in the middle of the forest all night as the father would walk away quietly, leaving the lad all alone. The father told him when he could see light through the blindfold, he could remove it...because it was now dawn. The first sign of light, the boy removed his blindfold and looked around... there just across from him...only feet away, was his father sitting there. His father had not left him all night, but had just sat there watching him till morn. The father told his son..."NOW YOU ARE A MAN"! The moral of the story went on to say that the same as this natural father sat and watched his son all night...our Father in heaven is keeping watch over us all night making sure we're safe from all harm. I cannot tell you the peace I felt after reading this message. Along with the CD that played peacefully while I was pushed through that space like capsule of an MRI, I imagined the Lord sitting on that stump keeping a watchful eye over me in the dark of night in that tube. I was then at peace. All went well with my MRI and I was so proud that I made it through. It was normally a 45 minute procedure that lasted well over an hour, but I just thank God it was all over.

Thursday June 19, 2008- This day was very painful for me. In addition to trying to absorb my learning of my cancer, Dr. Harland called to give me the test results from my MRI. I remember the call as though it were yesterday. She called at approximately 7:00 p.m. I was given the opportunity to come in for a face to face consultation or she could talk with me via phone. I chose the latter. Her voice was delightful as always. She went on to say, Althea, we have the results of your MRI. She explained medically how technology determines via satellites of light the detection of cancer cells. These satellites of light highlight areas of the organs that contain cancer cells. She explained that my tests showed satellites of light all in my left breast...so much so that there was no way to save the breast. She said further that my breast would need to be removed. I heard her but could not believe what she was saying. She explained that there was some indication in the right breast as well, but not of great concern as the left breast. She said we would revisit the right breast condition later. I remember quietly sobbing on the phone and begging if there was another way to save my breast... if there was another procedure to be done. I clearly wanted to know all my options. One is always advised to check your other options or get a second opinion on any medical diagnosis, especially a diagnosis as critically important as this one. I had full confidence in Dr. Harland. I valued her opinion and/or diagnosis in my case. However, I still felt a need to ask if there was any other way to proceed to aggressively combat this disease. She assured me that there was no other option and a mastectomy is highly recommended. She asked me if I was alright, and I just wanted to go into a room and just holler... scream...and....cry! I ended my call with her and experienced an emotional breakdown!

My daughter, Brittanie, my grand-daughters, Amaya, and Paul were all downstairs in our family room. I asked Paul, to come upstairs...I'd gone to my room where he followed. I just lost it! I was crying and screaming so loud...totally devastated. I could hardly tell him what the doctor said. Paul was trying desperately to figure out what I was saying through my tears. I struggled through my tears to tell him the news Dr. Harland told me. He could only hold me and allow me to cry. I told him to please get my granddaughter, Amaya, out of the house. I did not want her to see me so distraught. I believe Paul told Brittanie what had happened. She was in total shock! Brittanie was able to exit the house through the basement. Brittanie rushed Amaya out of the house, with her overnight bag in hand. Fortunately, Amaya didn't see me in such a traumatic state. Brittanie immediately put Amaya in the car and drove her to my church to her Mom, Dana. Dana was at church attending a youth function. I was such a horrible sight to see.

I could not believe my news...I had already received such terrible news in the past couple of weeks and this was more than I could handle. For the first time, I asked the Lord why was he doing this? He knew I had been so strong through this difficult time, but this latest news was more than enough. All I could do was cry and scream. Nothing relieved my pain.

Both my sisters, Evelyn and Lorraine, came over to my house after Paul called them to help try and console me. Evelyn prayed like I'd never heard her before. Lord did they pray for me! They encouraged me in every way they could. I began to hear both of them praying together with the sound of Evelyn's voice crying out to the Lord with such power. Their prayers consoled and comforted me, and made me feel much better. As suddenly as I'd felt the pain from receiving such horrible news, I felt calm and peace. Their prayers were really what I needed. Evelyn and Lorraine stayed awhile longer. We all sat around and had a nice sisterly chat and at times shared many laughs. We reminisced over our past, growing up, and remembered some of the most humorous moments. They finally had to leave. I really didn't want to see them go. They lifted my spirits…just what I needed.

My tears seemed to subside and the agony of it all silenced within a couple of hours. Later that evening, like waking up from a horrible nightmare, my tears began to flow again. Calmer than earlier that evening, I remember saying to myself…I have to get a grip on this and prayerfully seek the Lord on what I need to do. I decided that I have a husband, daughters, and grandbabies to live for and my life is worth more to me than my breasts. I had to come to that reality in my mind in order to move on from that moment. I then agreed to the mastectomy at whatever emotional cost it was to me. Paul agreed that that was best! We were at peace with our decision.

Friday, June 20, 2008-I had a consultation appointment with Dr. Norman Foster of Fairway Fayette Hospital. Dr. Foster was the Surgeon who would surgically place a port in my chest under my collar bone. Surgically placing a port in your chest gives access for chemotherapy treatment. The nurse technicians at GEORGIA CANCER CENTER injects a needle into the port as a source of entry intravenously for chemotherapy treatment. Lab work can be provided also by accessing a port. Everything was happening so fast at this point. All I could think of was my chest would now have to be cut open to place this device and I still hadn't accepted the fact that I had cancer. Would someone please stop this train?! I spoke with a Physician Assistant to Dr. Foster who thoroughly explained the surgery to me. He had me complete paperwork to take to my pre-op appointment which was to follow.

CHAPTER 6
THANK GOD FOR THE SUPPORT OF FAMILY AND FRIENDS "A CELEBRATION OF LOVE"

Sunday, June 22, 2008-This was such a fun day for me! Dana, Derron, Paul, Wanda (Derron's Mom), and Brittanie planned this big dinner for me. They knew that I would no longer be able to have company over to the house once the chemo treatment was started. The chemo would cause my immune system to become dangerously low, and I would not be able to interact with others. They prepared quite a barbecue feast. We had family and friends over. How nice it was. We ate, laughed, watched movies, and had a wonderful time! Dana and Brittanie gave me a surprise gift that really made my day.

Unaware to me during the dinner, they were passing around this cute little gift pillow that played the musical tune... *"He's got the Whole World in his Hands."* Everyone autographed this pillow with sweet words of encouragement. That sweet gesture helped me through this dark time. I could just press the pillow, play the music, and feel peace like never before.

Brittanie presented the pillow to me the following morning, just as I was getting ready to go to my first Oncologist visit.

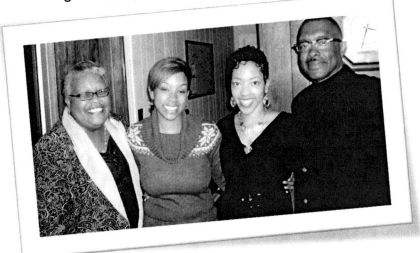

I cried so much, and could not stop comforting myself with it and playing the music. What a sweet and thoughtful gift. Brittanie insisted that Dana purchased it and it was all her idea. I was just so glad to have something to hold onto that would always remind me of the ones I loved. It was really a great day with family and friends!

CHAPTER 7

MY FIRST VISIT WITH MY ONCOLOGIST- A BATTERY OF SCANS AND TESTS

Monday, June 23, 2008-This was my very first visit to the Georgia Cancer Center office in Fayetteville under Dr. Sharian's care. I must say, when I walked into this office, I experienced a coldness that really troubled me. I looked on the faces of the people sitting in the waiting room. They had various expressions, some desperate, some lost, some pained, but many surprisingly were in cheerful spirits. I found that keeping a good positive attitude, during any illness, is the key to maintaining good health. So I immediately walked in with a smile, as only I can do, and greeted everyone warmly. With a kind smile, I'd hoped to somehow help cheer up those who seemed down. The front desk receptionist greeted me in the most professional way as I completed my paperwork, submitted my referral from my Primary Care Physician and insurance card. All seemed in order as I waited for my name to be called. First area of attention was my labs. This was my first stop each visit after signing in at the front desk. Two of the sweetest young ladies you ever want to meet were there waiting for me and treated me as though we were old girlfriends who knew each other years ago. Olivia and Helen...very charming nurses with so much personality! They made my very first visit a wonderful one. I felt I'd made two more friends who would help get me through a very tough and long journey. Each visit with them was showered with infectious laughter and kindness. This team of professionals knew exactly how to turn a depressing visit into a remarkably enjoyable one!

I was then taken back to Dr. Sharian's office by his delightful nurse, Molly. She was a joy to meet and always lovely to talk to. She too was a breast cancer survivor and my inspiration. Dr. Sharian came into his office and was as charming and warm, just as Dr. Harland had promised. I tell you, the Lord had placed all the doctors and medical professionals in my path that I needed. I found this overwhelming. Paul and Amaya were with me and both joined me for my doctor's consultation. Dr. Sharian was so accommodating and playful with Amaya. He told her that he has a daughter nearly her same age…4. Amaya returned his gesture of kindness and proceeded to read her books that we'd brought with her to keep her busy.

Dr. Sharian was very candid about my test results received from my biopsy. He concurred with Dr. Harland that the cancer in my left breast was malignant and the breast needed to be removed. He informed me of the type of cancer I had, that it was a stage 2 breast cancer. The findings from my MRI exam showed that the cancer was a fast growing cancer and had to be attacked aggressively. He recommended a weekly antibiotic treatment called Herceptin designed for women with HER2 Neu positive cancer that would be administered to me once a week for one year. This antibiotic acts as a blocker against the multiplying of cancer cells. He also recommended an infusion of two chemotherapy treatments, Carboplatin and Texotere to be administered every 3 weeks for 18 weeks. With all that was going on in preparation of all this treatment, I could only focus on November 2008 as my target date to complete this chemo madness. Once Dr. Sharian briefed me on the process, the diagnosis, the side effects, and all expectancies, he left us alone with Molly. Molly reviewed the various chemotherapy treatments with me. She gave us a lot of reading materials and answered our questions. She was quite thorough. Since she had gone through the illness as well, she was empathetic and comforting to talk to.

Molly then escorted us on a tour of their facility including the chemo treatment area. I remember not being able to look upon the faces of the patients receiving their treatments. I could only look away. I felt I'd invaded the privacy of those who had received the horrible news of cancer the same as I had. Like me, I thought they'd want to be left alone with their suffering. It was a pretty depressing encounter for me. The nurses were all very warm. I just wanted to get out of there! I was then escorted back to the front desk. Molly said goodbye and vowed to help make my time there with them very comfortable. She assured me that I would get through this. The ladies at the scheduling desk took quite a bit of time preparing my upcoming schedule of appointments. There was so much scheduling to do. I didn't realize how involved the scheduling process was. My appointments consisted of outside doctor's visits, multiple exams, and procedures, along with follow up appointments with Dr. Sharian. This was such an intense and time consuming visit ...unforgettable.

Monday, June 23, 2008- On this same day I had a bone scan scheduled just across the street from the GEORGIA CANCER CENTER facility at Fairway Fayette Hospital at 12:00 p.m. Once checking in with the hospital for my appointment, I was given an injection in the x-ray area. I was then asked to leave the area, drink plenty fluids and return at 3:00 that afternoon. Not realizing I had to spend all this time preparing for the procedure, Paul, Amaya and I left to go eat lunch. We spent time on the hospital grounds taking in the sights of the small lake and then went back for my procedure after 3 hours. The procedure took approximately 2 ½ hours and I was ready to go home. This was really an exhausting day!

Wednesday, June 25, 2008-I had an appointment on this day to see a Cardiologist in Newnan, Georgia by the name of Dr. Reid. At this office, the technicians would give me an ultrasound and echocardiogram. This would measure the health of my heart. It would ultimately determine if my heart was sound enough to withstand chemotherapy treatment. All of the tests I'd taken leading up to my taking the chemo treatments would determine whether or not my organs and body was sound enough for treatment. Each test was vitally important. I am learning so much from the Lord each day of this journey. One thing I've learned that is so important, to be attentive to every single individual that comes into your life. Furthermore, it is imperative to keep your spiritual ears open to hear when the Lord speaks through each individual. One never knows how the Lord will speak through or use them. The nurse technician who performed my tests was very instrumental in introducing me to a product that I believed would help serve as a catalyst in my healing.

The technician was very nice. We had the best conversation during the course of my examination. She began to share with me that her husband was a 3 year throat cancer survivor, and he'd never even been a smoker. I was amazed to hear this. She stated that reports are being revealed everyday of cases where people develop throat cancer without ever being a cigarette smoker or using nicotine. She continued to tell me how he received his treatment and cure at a Cancer Treatment Center in Texas. She then suggested a product for me to look into and start using. That was my first time hearing about it and I was fascinated. This juice product is an all natural vitamin supplement that supplies daily servings of fruits and vegetables. I learned later after getting back home, that Paul was very familiar with this product. The technician said this product has been proven by extensive research to cure Prostate Cancer. She began to conclude that if it cures Prostate Cancer, certainly it will cure other forms of cancer. She went on to explain all the great benefits of this juice product, and how it, along with exercise, had revitalized her husband's life. After my exam with the technician, I left with a promise that I would keep her husband in my prayers and she would remember me in hers. It was a great visit. I really enjoyed our conversation. I saw the Lord in every step of my journey and in everyone I met. It was simply amazing!

Wednesday, June 25, 2008- On this same day, I had an appointment with the GEORGIA CANCER CENTER for a CT scan. For this procedure I had to drink a barium sulfate solution 6 hours prior to my appointment. My appointment with GEORGIA CANCER CENTER was 1:30 p.m. so I was rushing earlier that morning to get this entire solution down before the clock struck 7:30 a.m.! (smile) It wasn't bad and I got it all done. In addition to drinking this solution, I couldn't eat or drink anything until after my CT scan. By the time I left the Cardiologist's office and got to the GEORGIA CANCER CENTER, I was getting pretty hungry. I walked into the GEORGIA CANCER CENTER and guess what they have waiting for me when I get there…another round of barium sulfate to drink. I wasn't sure what this stuff was

supposed to do before a CT scan, but I would certainly have a stomach full of it before my exam! (smile) I finished the solution...once again, and they called me back to prepare for my CT scan. I have the worst veins in the world when injecting needles for IV's, so my upcoming port surgery will be a welcoming transition from being poked so many times for IV injections. To say the least, this technician had the hardest time finding a good vein in my arm to inject the saline solution. After a couple of tries, with no success, she injects my hand (how I hated to have the back of my hand injected with a needle).
Later, a dye was inserted to give the test a good read. Thank God, I thought, now let's get on with this scan! The technician was so friendly and worked skillfully to complete the test. Once the test was done, all I wanted to do was get out of there to go find something to eat. I was famished!

Thursday, June 26, 2008-I had an appointment for pre-op services at Fairway Fayette Hospital in preparation for my port insertion surgery that was scheduled for July 1st. This was another day of meeting people who the Lord would place in my path for me to minister to or who would minister to me. The first admissions clerk that I met was a beautiful young lady who really loved the Lord. Her heart went out to me in my condition. I was rather emotional this day, as I've been most days since learning of my illness. This young lady began to minister to me and encourage me in the Lord. She shared scriptures of power that spoke healing into my life. I could see that she was a true Christian as I was. My emotions got the best of me this day and all I could do was acknowledge the Lord's voice through her. How amazing to meet and hear God's people at a time in your life when you really need them. She began to tell me while she's preparing my paperwork for admission and placing an arm bracelet on my arm, about her ministry at her church. She shared with me about many members in her church, who were cancer survivors. She also told me how these members had shared their stories with others and witnessed God's awesome healing power in their lives. We began to exchange phone numbers, and e-mail addresses. She promised to pray for me, have her church pray for me, and would have one of her Ministers call me. I so looked forward to hearing from her and her church members. We both acknowledged that our churches have the same spirit of prayer and share a powerful move of God. She was truly another angel that the Lord placed in my path. I cannot stress enough the importance of paying attention to everyone the Lord places in your life...especially on your journey through dark times.

I then went on to the nurse who took my vital signs, completed extensive forms of questions concerning my present meds, verified my medical history, and updated my present medical records in preparation for surgery. She finally instructed me on everything I needed for surgery. My surgery was scheduled for July 1, 2008. She answered any questions that I had. I was then free to leave and report back for surgery on 7/1.
I left the hospital feeling very prepared for what I was about to face. They made me feel very confident about the entire procedure.

CHAPTER 8
HOW SAD TO LEAVE MY JOB IF ONLY FOR AWHILE

Thursday, June 26, 2008- I was nearing the end of my work schedule; preparing to leave my job on short term disability leave. My co-workers planned this surprise going away party for me that I really was in no mood for. I wanted to leave graciously, yet express my love and appreciation for what they wanted to do for me. I'm not the kind of person who welcomes a lot of attention to oneself. I am a shy person when it comes to that kind of thing. I love celebrating and honoring others…not myself. Considering my emotional state at that point in my life with the discovery of my illness and having to leave work so suddenly, I did not want a celebration to bring more attention to that. It was hard enough to leave my job...having a party and saying goodbye would be even more difficult. I really enjoyed my job, working alongside some of the most wonderful people. Respecting my feelings, instead, they all decided to revise the party plans. The staff had all gotten together and personalized the most thoughtful gifts for me. Ann Collins, our Vice-President of Program called me into her office by mid-afternoon, closed the door, and said she had something for me from EVERYONE in the office. Ann presented it to me in a stunning *"Red breast cancer survivor inspirational tote bag"* (she said she looked for a pink bag but couldn't find one). Man, this bag was an original! How touched I was. First of all she presented me with the most gorgeous red tote bag that was personally autographed by everyone in the office. The bag was embossed with classic designs including the beautiful breast cancer pink ribbon emblem. There were also colorful daisies glued onto the bag. How original and enlightening. The bag contained gifts that were personalized by each co-worker and it expressed their own personalities. Ann shared every single gift with me and told me who it was from. I received a replica of ballet shoes from one co-worker who was a dancer;

the cross of David; a St Christopher Catholic necklace (that promised to always protect), a New Orleans Saints necklace from one of my co-workers that was a rival to our Atlanta Falcons; a wonderful Spanish CD from Ann's husband's group; along with a crystal jewel piece that she said would clearly help me see into my future. Also included were inspirational books, CD's, friendship plaques, and various lotions. I was never so touched. I promised to take that bag with me to each one of my chemo treatment visits and think of my co-workers every moment that I needed inspiration.

Friday, June 27, 2008-This is my last day at work and boy did I have a lot of loose ends to tie up. I was most happy that this was a day of "no doctor's appointments or exams." I could focus only on work and what I needed to do before I left on disability leave. It was so emotional for me. This was a very difficult time in my life. Everything was happening so fast. I worked so hard and packed up as much as I could for the time I would be away. I also wanted to prepare my work space for whom ever would replace me for the time I would be out. I stayed and worked until nearly 8:00 that evening. Lisa Jordan, the President of our company, was still working as we said our goodbyes in the parking lot. It was heartfelt and so hard to tell her goodbye.

I knew I'd be back soon, but at that moment it felt like it would be a lifetime. She was so kind and concerned. She asked me to let her know if there was anything she could do for me. I was touched and we went our separate ways. My final moments would be spent with our Security team at work, Michael and Tim. They were the finest and nicest two young men. They helped me transport all my personal belongings and boxes to my car. We stood out in the parking lot and chatted humorously for awhile. They promised to keep in touch and come out to visit me when I felt up to it. We hugged and I left, oh how my heart ached!

CHAPTER 9
THE DELIGHT OF MEETING NEW FRIENDS-I GET MY FIRST WIG!

Saturday, June 28, 2008-This was a delightful day. I had the wonderful opportunity to meet some of Paul's friends he'd met while working on his last job in Tallapoosa, Georgia. They were Sally and Bill Moss. They were the kindest people. Bill was a long-time mechanic who would rescue Paul from automotive problems on the highway… more times than he can count. Paul and Bill were Vietnam buddies as well. They'd built a bond that was very special. Bill and Sally owned a Health Food store in the area. Paul would periodically purchase health food items, vitamins, and supplements from her. This day we went, not only to meet them, but to place an order for the juice product that I learned about. Sally had a vast knowledge of the product along with testimonials of how it helped heal Bill of a severe heart condition. We were all ears and could not believe some of the cures of cancer and various health issues that this product helped. We placed our order and visited with them awhile. One of the highlights of my visit was to meet Sally's Mom, Mrs. Hanson. She was a devout praying Christian woman that anyone would love to meet. Her warm embrace and smile seemed to have healed my body while sitting there with her. She encouraged me in the Word of the Lord and asked me to rely on my faith in God for my healing. Our visit was short with Mrs. Hanson but remarkably memorable. Sally and Bill prayed with us before we left, as Mrs. Hanson had to get back to her home up the street to her grands and great grandchildren. Sally's prayer moved me in a way that I really needed. I would not soon forget Mrs. Hanson, Sally, Bill, their grandchildren and family. We left there knowing that we had friends who would last a lifetime. How much I needed this visit!

Saturday, June 28, 2008-After leaving Sally and Bill I had another extraordinary visit with an old friend from my church. Andrea Davis was more than a friend, she was like family. She was my original hairdresser when I came to Atlanta. She relocated to Washington, D.C. but visits the city periodically. She is also dear friends with my Pastors' family. It was Andreas' gift to me, during my illness, to purchase my very first wig to wear in preparation for my hair loss from the chemo. She met me in the parking lot of my church and we went to a nearby wig shop that another friend of mine owned. There were at least 4 showrooms of wigs to shop from. How fascinating that was! What impressed me the most with Andrea is that not only did she want to bless me with this gift, but the time and patience that she took with me to make sure that I chose the right wig for my face. After all, she was a professional beautician and an expert! We spent it seemed like hours in that shop. She had a chance to meet Sandra, my girlfriend who owned the shop. Andrea had this infectious personality that anyone she meets falls in love with her humor and candor. She was opinionated about everything and only settles for perfection. I loved it! Immediately she had the attention of all the girls in the shop and had them all at her service! What was so empathetic about Andrea's kindness is that she is a Leukemia survivor and has also suffered an Aneurysm in her life. Her extraordinary love of people and desire to give herself to others is a testament of who she is as a person.

I loved her expression of love to me when I needed it most! We made our final selections and I walked out of the shop with an awesome wig from Andrea, along with one from Sandra, the owner. I would look like a *"Diva"* even if I didn't feel like one. How impressed I was...and they really made me feel much better!

CHAPTER 10
DISAPPOINTING NEWS- A RESCHEDULE OF MY FIRST DAY OF CHEMOTHERAPY

Monday, June 30, 2008-This was the day that I thought would be my first day of chemotherapy treatment. I went to the Georgia Cancer Center in such fear. I cannot tell you how scared I was. I checked in, completed my routine paperwork at the front desk; and then went back for my labs. One of the nurses, Philippe, who prepared me for my labs impressed me immensely. He was a very serious young man and totally competent. He gave me my IV injection to administer my chemo. He was the nurse I complimented above all. He took blood from me my very first day at GEORGIA CANCER CENTER

(6/23/08), and amazingly enough, I did not feel any pain or pinch from his poke in my vein as I have from all other blood work sticks that I've received. It had been quietly herald that he had this reputation around the lab office... that if Philippe can't find your veins, NOBODY in the office could...so he was the best! In my mind, he was very special. The fact that he was done sticking me, and taking my blood before I ever even noticed was remarkable. I was still waiting for him to stick me...and it was all over. How wonderful. However, unfortunately for me, on this particular day, he came into the office to take my labs from injecting my IV, and he could not find a vein ANYWHERE in my arm. He was even shocked. But to his credit, I quickly told him that I had been stuck so many times in my right arm in the past 3 weeks that I don't think my veins would respond to ANYONE at this point! (smile) My right arm was always the arm used for all lab work, due to the fact that the cancer was located in my left breast. I was told that due to medical concerns, my left arm should never be used to draw blood or any lab work. Using the arm on the side of my breast that contained cancer could cause lymph edema and swelling of the glands. This can prove to be detrimental to one's health. My right arm became over exhausted and needed a rest from all my upcoming doctor visits! (smile)

I then went back to see Dr. Sharian. He realized that I would have my port surgery the following morning, so he decided to cancel any chemo treatment and move it to the following Monday, July 7th. This way, it would give my port time to heal. I was somewhat relieved. At least when I came back for my first chemo treatment, I would have my port in place and NEVER have to worry about being stuck in my arm or hand EVER again! THANK YOU LORD!

Monday, June 30, 2008- Since my first chemo treatment was cancelled I decided to go on back home to wait for my next appointment which was scheduled for 1:45 that same afternoon. Paul and I decided to go on home and come back later. We would have had to wait nearly 3 hours for the PET scan appointment. I came back for a PET scan scheduled at the Epicure PET of Fayetteville that afternoon. After going to doctors' offices all across the city; I thought how convenient. Their office was located just across the street from the cancer center office and provided a professional, friendly team of nurses. After completing routine paperwork and insurance requirements, they escorted me to the back where I was injected with yet another IV in my arm. Through this IV, they inserted dye to administer a PET scan. The dye was used to give clear view of organs that might be affected with cancer. Once the dye was inserted into my vein, I had to lie down for one hour before my test could be performed in order for the dye to properly circulate. Once in the x-ray room, I was placed on a table, similar to the bone and CT scan procedures. I found the PET scan procedure to be long and at times uncomfortable. I had to lie on a table in pretty tight quarters while being mobilized slowly through this machine. At times the movement would be meticulously slow and I would have to hold my body in one position for very long periods of time. I found this position to be very uncomfortable. Nevertheless, I made it through and I was SO glad that this test too was over. I found the PET scan procedure tame compared to the MRI! (smile) How I prayed ALL these tests would end so I could go back to somewhat of a normal day.

Tuesday, July 1, 2008-Well, with all the doctor appointments, exams and tests leading up to my first chemotherapy treatment, I am finally ready to have my port surgery. Again, I go back to Fairway Fayette Hospital for outpatient surgery. My reporting for surgery and preparation for it went pretty smoothly and quickly. Due to the difficulty of finding veins to insert an IV for anesthesia, the nurse finally had to insert the IV in my inner wrist. How painful and uncomfortable that was. I remember saying to myself…how long is this surgery?! I don't know how long I will be able to endure this discomfort in my inner wrist. However, I also felt some relief, since I knew this would be my last time having a needle in my arm, wrist, or hand. That was a relief!

I remember Dr. Foster coming in the room before I was taken to surgery to say hello and make sure I was alright. He assured me that everything would be just fine. I rested in his kind reassurance. The Anesthesiologist came in to inject anesthesia into my IV. I remembered being in surgery and hearing the voice of the Surgeon asking if I was alright and if I was feeling any pain. I shook my head letting him know that I wasn't. They assured me that I was doing well and they were almost done. I could hear the Surgeon giving instructions to other medical personnel in the room as well. I was then taken back to the initial room I was in before surgery. There, another nurse came in, checked vital signs, monitored my progress, removed my IV, gave me pain medication and prescriptions, and finally had me sign release forms. She clarified any final care instructions that she needed to review with me and answered any questions I had.

When I was completely alert, she kindly placed me in a wheelchair and wheeled me to the exit doors while Paul went to get our car from the parking lot to take me home. That part of my process was finally over!

CHAPTER 11
SECOND BIOPSY- FOLLOW UP FROM MY PET SCAN (SUSPICIOUS CELLS)

Thursday July 3, 2008-Well, it's the day before the 4th of July holiday and everyone's preparing picnic and cookout celebrations, while I'm recuperating from surgery. I am quite sore and trying to find a good sleeping position without discomfort. The pain medication prescribed does the trick and I thank God for relief. This is also the day that I go to the Breast Cancer Care office to have my biopsy procedure done on my right breast. My previous MRI showed satellite lights in the right breast as well as my left. While they didn't suspect a problem in the right breast, they wanted to take precautions to have an ultrasound done on it. At this point all these painful procedures seemed like too much to handle in that they were scheduled so close together. I was becoming so exhausted and frustrated with SO many exams and tests. I went in to have the ultrasound done. After the technician completed the test she asked me to relax until the Radiologist reviewed the results. I laid there thinking and praying for the best. So much was going through my mind at this time. All I could think about was what would these results show? Up to this point in this whole journey, I'd received nothing but bad news…I just couldn't take more. It was in the hands of the Lord at this point. Please God…I prayed…no more bad news!

The Radiologist, Dr. Spencer, comes back into the room, along with two technicians and gives me my results. Apparently, the ultrasound could not give her a conclusive report of the mass that the original MRI showed. She then said the words that I dreaded to hear…I'd have to go back through another MRI exam. The MRI machine is my fear above all fears throughout this entire process and succession of tests. There's no way I could go back through that again…GOD NO…PLEASE! I suddenly became claustrophobic with just the thought of going through that procedure again. I hyperventilated just thinking about going back through this dark tunnel again! I lay there on the table hearing Dr. Spencer's words with tears of desperation. She sees my fear and watches me cry. She immediately went into *calm mode*. She tried easing my fears of the machine, its purpose, as well as its benefits. She emphasized the fact that I need to come to grips with the MRI machine. She said I need to embrace the machine as my friend and realize that it will be the best indicator to measure the progress and/or status of my cancer.

I then asked if Paul could come into the room from the waiting area so she could explain her findings with him. She agreed and the nurses went out to get Paul and Amaya so that Dr. Spencer could consult with him. Paul saw I was upset and tried also to calm me down. She explained to him that she had to perform the biopsy during the MRI exam in order to clearly see the proper site that needed biopsying. She also explained in great detail the entire process and what would be done. This procedure would take longer than the initial 45 minute MRI process that I previously endured. My nerves were shot! Just the thought of the length of time I would have to be in that dreadful capsule horrified me!

Dr. Spencer then scheduled an appointment for me to come back for an MRI biopsy procedure to take place on July 10th. I had the holiday weekend to pray and prepare myself for another experience with the terrifying MRI machine. Of course, once again, I would be medicated to go through this procedure. Thank God for medicating fears!(smile)

Thursday, July 3, 2008-On this same day I had an appointment with my Gynecologist, Dr. Donald Yancey. This appointment was set up as a result of a referral via Dr. Sharian after my PET scan (6/30/08) revealed a fibroid mass on my uterus and a cyst on my ovaries. Dr. Sharian was very concerned about the possibility of cancer cells contained in these masses since cancer is known to spread to other parts of the body. Dr. Sharian further revealed that there was a spot seen on my lung as well. He did not seem to have great concern about the spot on my lung. It was very small in size.

This discovery shot my blood pressure back up very high. I knew I could not take any more bad news. That seemed to be all the news I was getting since I learned of my cancer. GOD PLEASE, NO MORE BAD NEWS! Dr. Sharian prepared a CD of these findings on film to take to Dr. Yancey's office.

Dr. Yancey talked candidly with both Paul and me about what the PET scan test results showed. He scheduled an ultrasound of his own in his office. He scheduled it for the following week to see what it showed. He simply wanted to administer his own test, get the results immediately, and go from there. Paul and I took this time to discuss the discovery of my cancer with him. Paul was very angry about my being diagnosed with cancer, when he knew I kept an impeccable record of annual checkups and stayed abreast of my health issues.

He had many questions as to why my mammogram a year ago didn't reveal that I had breast cancer and to the degree that it showed…stage 2. Dr. Yancey discussed several diagnosis and prognosis that could or could not have shown the cancer cells. It was his medical and professional opinion that the cancer cells could have been there a year ago, but sometimes mammograms do not show these findings until sometime later. He thoroughly explained the nature of cancer cells and how they can lie dormant in the body and are sometimes, not readily detected via mammogram technology. We were just devastated that this discovery was not revealed to us earlier.

CHAPTER 12

"INDEPENDENCE DAY"- A CELEBRATION AND TIME OF RELAXATION WITH MY DAUGHTER (WHAT FUN!)

Friday, July 4, 2008-It's the 4th of July; A day of celebration and fun for millions of Americans as we mark the day of our country's independence! However, the Lord woke me up early this holiday morning with such a joyous spirit. In spite of all that I'd been through and the pain of it all, the Lord was speaking to me to encourage me and say… "this day will not be a sad one for you." "This is the day that I, the Lord has made, and you will rejoice and be glad in it!" I was suddenly so excited about the day and what was to come! We didn't have any celebration plans in store, no fireworks, sparkles, or festivities. I was just glad to be alive and happy to know that I had my family with me and people who I knew loved me. And that's all that mattered. I was determined to make this a fun-filled day!

I really wanted to go later that day, visit my daughter Dana, and stay at her place for the weekend. Her place proved to be a peaceful getaway for me for the weekend. I could rest, relax, and let my mind not worry about my condition or what I had to go through the upcoming week. My day started off with an inspirational visit from the Lord and a powerful prayer. My goddaughter, Misty and her brother, Jason, came by the house to pay me a surprise visit. It was so good to see them and such perfect timing. Misty is the kind of person who would not allow anyone around her to be sad or depressed. She immediately asked me to get up, get dressed, and enjoy the day! She would not take no for an answer. Paul and Jason went outside to visit with our dogs, German Shepherds, who are trained in Schutzhund training.

Jason told us how he longed to own a German Shepherd puppy. His Mom, however, who he is now living with, would not allow it. We tried to encourage him to convince his Mom to agree to a puppy. They are such wonderful and genuinely protective dogs. That brought such a laugh to all us trying to convince Jason to change his Mom's mind. Misty and Jason had to leave to get back home to their own family cookout. They invited us to come as well, but we had to refuse. We'd already made plans to go spend the day and weekend with Dana at her place. We shared hugs and kisses then they left. They didn't realize how their visit added such enjoyment to the beginning of my day!

Dana reminded us that she had chicken in her freezer from an earlier cookout that we had weeks ago. She offered to add that to a cookout her boyfriend, Derron would host at his place. I added some *"fixins"* from my refrigerator along with condiments, utensils and picnic supplies. We were on our way to her place for a fun afternoon. Derron is a master grilling King…and we always enjoy his succulent texture of grilled meats and corn. Our mouths watered as we prepared ourselves to feast. We ate good, laughed, watched movies, and had a great day. I really needed that!

Paul left to go on back home, while Brittanie, Dana, Amaya and I went on home with Dana to her place to prepare for a very relaxing evening and weekend. Dana continually said how happy she was to have me stay at her place. She had no idea, she could not have been happier than me! Amaya was just as excited to have Grandma stay with her...even sleep in her bed. Dana's apartment served as a place of refuge for me away from all my cares and worries. It was the perfect idea for my weekend getaway. Paul and I wanted to go to Midway Gardens for the holiday weekend to get away, however our finances could not accommodate us. Dana's place really sufficed beyond our dreams. I was so happy to be there. I spent quality time with Dana, Brittanie, and Amaya. Brittanie got dressed to go out with some of her friends that evening. She kissed me goodbye and promised me she would call me Saturday morning before she went to work. I'm always the concerned

Mom, and made her promise me she would call me when she got home that night.

Amaya and I played and toured her beautiful bedroom. Her bedroom was a Disney wonderland of Princesses from Cinderella to Jasmine. It was a most delightful sight. I have visited her bedroom on many occasions but she always treats me like a first time guest! (smile) She was always so excited to share her dream bedroom. We watched a little television, talked, laughed and ate a late night snack. We then all retired for bed.

Saturday July 5, 2008- I am always the early riser in the house. I awoke early that morning, prayed and went online on Dana's laptop to check e-mails. It's always nice to check e-mail messages from my family and friends. They kept me encouraged and entertained. Dana and Amaya later awakened, and again Amaya and I played. Dana and I talked and caught up on what was going on in her life.
She always welcomed my Motherly advice. It was such a great visit. We planned to go to a special park I loved near her home on the lake. It was such a

peaceful scenic spot. This park had become a favorite spot of mine. Along the lake were ducks, geese, and boaters who were also enjoying the holiday weekend. The lake was so relaxing. My mind was at peace and I was able to collect my thoughts and quietly look forward to my upcoming week. I could not ask for anything more! Amaya and Dana played on the playground where I later went to join them. We enjoyed ourselves. It was so much fun…then we left to go home. I would not forget the images of the park and its restful rewards.

When we returned to Dana's home, we watched a DVD of one of her favorite gospel artists, **"Israel and New Breed"**. It was one of the most anointed performances of ministry that I'd seen. The DVD showed the essence of their ministry. Each minister and singer spoke about what the name **"New Breed"** meant and what ministry meant to them. They further expressed what the anointing meant to them and what they vowed to accomplish in their effort to minister each time they performed. I thoroughly enjoyed this DVD. We then began to play a variety of gospel praise and worship songs. We had a great time in the Lord...just havin' church! I played one CD that Brittanie prepared for me. This CD had the most powerful praise and worship songs that I'd ever heard ministered. I really wanted to share this worship experience with Dana. The entire atmosphere in the apartment was one of anointed worship. For that one moment in time, we both forgot about all our cares and allowed the Lord's anointing to resonate within our spirits...it blessed us immensely.

How fresh and spiritually fulfilled we felt. I looked over at Dana and she was in tears and so was I! What a moment with the Lord and my daughter. After we came back down to earth from our heavenly experience, we then put on some shout music! Amaya led us in the shout and we had a Holy Ghost good time in the Lord right in her living room. We made sure that her neighbor wasn't at home below her apartment. He wasn't, so we commenced to let the Lord have His way in our lives. I mean we really let it RIP! (smile) All three of us, Dana, Amaya and I just shouted our heads off! What a good time we had! (smile)

Dana wanted to spend the evening with Derron for a movie night. So I had Amaya all to myself to play, watch movies, and have fun. And we did. We played and watched movies until Dana returned home by early evening. Amaya was so excited to see her Mommy! Dana planned to go to church the following morning and I asked to let Amaya stay home with me so I could have a final day of fun with her before I left to go home that afternoon. She decided to let Amaya stay home with me. I was still unable to go to church. I was still recovering from my surgery.

Sunday, July 6, 2008- Dana arose early that morning preparing for church and I was already up...I'm the early bird! Dana wanted to say a prayer with me before she left for church. We assembled in the living room, our place of worship, for prayer. Lord knows she prayed the most anointed prayer ever! I cried, she cried, and we just knew the Lord heard our prayer. She prayed for healing, wholeness, and answered prayer to many requests we both have had before the Lord. The Lord used her mightily. I was still somewhat sore in my chest from my port surgery. When Dana went to hug me after her prayer, she gave me a bear hug like none other. I didn't want to tell her, but I was hurting so bad I almost saw stars! She had no idea that her huge hug was right on the side of my surgery. Nevertheless, I loved that moment. A peace came over my spirit like never before. How awesome!

After she left for church, Amaya and I played and had a wonderful Sunday morning together. We then prepared dinner…what fun! The night before, we all went shopping at Watkins and purchased fried chicken to supplement our Sunday dinner. Amaya and I simply opened canned beans, corn, Hawaiian sweet rolls, and soft drink. Amaya was so glad to help out in the kitchen, if only setting the table, opening up a can of veggies and doing her part. She is the greatest "*Grandma helper*"! We carefully planned the preparation timing of dinner to have it fresh and ready for Dana when she got home from church. When Dana got home, we were all so excited to see her, as though we hadn't seen her all day. It was just a fun day and weekend for me!

I suddenly became very sad.   The day was quickly coming to an end and I knew it meant that Paul was coming to pick me up to take me back home. I was saddened by the minute…just knowing that my *"perfectly relaxing"* weekend would end. I had imagined   that I was away at a very nice resort…Midway Gardens! (smile)   Leaving Dana's apartment and going back to my home only symbolized my leaving a peaceful environment and going back to a memory of all the pain and bad news of this cancer scare. Going back home meant preparing for the upcoming doctor appointments, frightening tests, lab work, and oh yes, chemo treatment.   Of course, going home to Paul was a joy. He and Brittanie had been the best support I could have ever asked for. They both seemed to know intimately what I needed. They knew when I wanted to talk and when I didn't. More importantly, they knew when I wanted to be alone and when I longed for their touch. They were the best. My, how my heart pounded as the time grew nearer and I had to leave…I can't tell you how much!

Paul arrived and ate dinner with us. Dana prepared a plate for Derron and we enjoyed our last moments together. Amaya had no idea what her Grandmommy was getting ready to undergo in the midst of all the playtime, fun, and sharing that we enjoyed all weekend. I stayed in high spirits for her, but Dana knew that it would be hard for me to leave. We packed up all my stuff and I prepared to leave. It was harder than I ever imagined. I cried from the time I left the apartment, as I slowly went down the stairway, and when I got into my car. I hugged Amaya so hard and Dana even harder. Dana knew the pain I felt. I remember putting my sunglasses on so that Amaya and Dana could not see how hard I was crying. I felt I would breathe my last breath. When I got in the car with Paul, he could not say anything. He knew how hard it was for me. He only sat quietly and allowed me to cry. The tears turned out to be so therapeutic for me. I could actually feel myself at the point of intense tears; then a sudden relief of soft sniffles followed. But as I would think of home, the intense tears came back all over again.

Paul had to stop by Tanners to pick up a solution to go in the water in our Jacuzzi to clean out our tub and the jets. He wanted to make a nice clean bubble bath for me to relax in when I got home. You see, he always knew what I needed and when I needed it! How intuitive of him. He was the best! While Paul went in the store, I sat in the car with a powerfully anointed song on a CD playing entitled, *"In God There Is No Failure."* The lyrics went on to say... *"He can do whatever you ask Him to."* I played that song repeatedly while he was gone. It ministered so incredibly to my spirit. The next thing I knew, my tears had miraculously dried up...so amazingly! Paul and I chatted all the way home about my weekend, and when I realized it, we were home and I didn't feel the agonizing pain that I was sure I would. I actually felt relieved to be home!

The Lord knows just how to minister to us, if we only let Him. It can come through a song, the whisper of a child, or through ducks in the park. He is an amazing God!

CHAPTER 13

MY SECOND RESCHEDULING TO START FIRST DAY OF CHEMOTHERAPY

Monday, July 7, 2008- We went to GEORGIA CANCER CENTER thinking again that this would be my very first chemo treatment and/or injection of Herceptin. I went in routinely to the lab area for the nurses to check my weight, labs, and inject my port with the saline solution that would initialize the injection of the Herceptin. I'm all prepared with a needle in my port and ready to receive the Herceptin treatment. Fortunately for me after going in first to see Dr. Sharian, he prepared to update me on my status. He immediately realized after checking his records that I had not had the biopsy ordered on my right breast. He became mildly annoyed with me. Apparently, as a result of a misunderstanding, on my part, I failed to follow his instructions. He needed the biopsy done on my right breast with results in hand before I could undergo ANY chemo treatments. I was supposed to make this appointment with BREAST CANCER CENTER and Dr. Spencer…and I hadn't. Dr. Sharian again reiterated as he did to me before, he did not want to go forward with chemo treatment before knowing conclusively that the cells in the right breast were not cancerous. The MRI biopsy would answer that question for him. I clearly remembered him saying that I needed to have the biopsy done first, but I had to undergo so many procedures and tests, I think my mind was completely exhausted. I missed this very important procedure before coming to his office for this appointment. I made a trip on this day that I should not have made. I had the lab nurses puncture my port in preparation for treatment that never should have been done. Everyone, including the lab nurses, chemotherapy nurses, and front desk saw and felt my disappointment in not starting my treatment. Who would've ever guessed that one could be so disappointed in not starting chemotherapy treatment?

Dr. Sharian sent me out of his office to go back to the front desk to reschedule the treatment AFTER I'd undergone the MRI biopsy on my right breast. I don't have to remind you that this procedure is the one that I dreaded more than ANY! Maybe the mental block was my fear of this test and subconsciously blocking the fact that I inadvertently placed the test after the treatment, and it clearly should have been taken before. Who knew, all I knew was that I walked away from that office feeling so disappointed.
My God, I thought, please place me on a clear path of healing in this journey. I was so tired of all these tests…especially the test that I feared most in life! I walked away and rode all the way home in tears…trying not to let Paul see.

CHAPTER 14

MY SECOND MRI- MORE ANXIETY!

Thursday, July 10, 2008-Well this is the day of my second MRI accompanied with a biopsy that would be performed on my right breast. This would be a most intense and painful day for me. You know the fear I already felt for the MRI and to have a biopsy procedure as well was more than my mind could take. I got to the Breast Cancer Center office for an 11:00 a.m. appointment at 10:15 a.m. As I've mentioned before, I must take my medication to relax me for the procedure ½ hour before the actual procedure is performed. I took my medication in my car as Paul and I drove up to the office. I wanted to make sure I was calm before I had to go through this.

I dressed in my gown, sat back in the waiting area outside the MRI office and waited and waited, for what seemed like an hour. A young lady came out of the office who was also a patient completely dressed, and she said they are having to cancel all appointments due to the malfunctioning of one of the machines. I thought, no not another disappointment and prolonging of time for something I need to get done and out of the way...PLEASE GOD NO! By now, I'm really getting upset that no one from the office bothered to come out and tell me what was going on or what happened.

Finally, shortly after the young lady told me they had to cancel all appointments one of the nurses did come out to tell me. She asked me to come back into the MRI area where she formerly told me what had happened. I believe there was some kind of electrical problem. She asked if they could reschedule me for later that afternoon, could I come back? Well, by now, I'm feeling pretty woozy from the medication and was concerned if Dr. Harland could call in another dose of it to my pharmacy for the rescheduled appointment time. She said she could, and would make all the arrangements. Paul and I left the office to go back home with a promise from them that they would call me back when the machinery was up and ready to go. My home is nearly a 35-40 minute drive from the Breast Cancer Care office, so we would have to double back, possibly in rush hour traffic to make it back for a second appointment.

Well, at 2:00 p.m., we received the call from the same nurse to come back for a 4:00 p.m. appointment, if possible. Knowing how important this test was for the onset of my chemo treatments, I immediately asked Paul if he could run by the pharmacy and pick up my prescription. I took the meds again and headed back to the Breast Care center. I would be one "drugged up camper" by the end of the day! (smile)

Wouldn't you guess…we got tied up in pouring rain with traffic on the interstate backed up for miles, we knew we wouldn't make it to this appointment by 4:00 p.m. as scheduled. When we saw that the rain would not stop and the traffic was moving to a crawl, we called the center at approximately 3:30 p.m. and told them we were running very late and may not be able to make it until 4:30 p.m. or possibly 4:45 that afternoon. They were so gracious and said to come on, they would wait for me. I knew they too knew how important this appointment and procedure was to me.

Dr. Spencer, who was the Radiologist and doctor who would perform the procedure, was right there waiting for me. We arrived at the center at exactly 4:45 with all patients gone home for the day. We walked right in, prepped for the procedure and it must have taken all of 2 hours for it to be completed. It had to be the most excruciatingly painful experience I've had, mentally, emotionally, and physically.

The technicians kept telling me to lie still (so hard to do after being in this contraption for 2 hours). Then I had to get pulled out of the machine for Dr. Spencer to perform the biopsy. How painful that was, even with local anesthesia. The last time I'm pushed back into the machine, I was instructed to hold my breath for more times than I could remember, and that was so very uncomfortable. Periodically holding your breath is normal procedure for this test.
This helps assure accurate x-rays. They began to tell me to hold on just a little longer. By now, I was gasping for air and found the procedure now

unbearable. Finally, they were done and they pulled me out. I could feel myself hyperventilating and needing air. I even became sick to my stomach, but managed to get to the restroom with the nurses' help before causing an accident on myself. I was so dazed from the medication I took before the procedure.

By this time, it's 7:10 in the evening. Once again, I could only breathe a sigh of relief that this was all over...and there was no need to repeat this procedure anytime soon. We left the office so exhausted and all I wanted again...WAS TO GO HOME! I believe I slept that entire night with all loss of time.

CHAPTER 15

A BREAK FROM THE MADNESS- A HAIR APPOINTMENT AND VISIT TO TV 5 STUDIOS

Tuesday, July 15, 2008-This day was by far one of my most exciting days of all. Brittanie and I first of all treated ourselves to a nice hair appointment with my hairdresser, Lexi and boy did she have us looking good! It would serve as my last hair appointment before losing my hair. It was very emotional for me, but Lexi made my visit an enjoyable one. She tried not to remind me of the hair I would lose, she only wanted to console me with the new hair cut she could give me once my hair grew back, and still keep me looking like a *"Diva"*! I liked that…who wouldn't?!

After leaving the salon, Brittanie wanted to take me to the TV 5 Studio to meet her co-workers, celebrity reporters, and others. She worked as a summer News Intern. As excited as I was for her and wanting to make this visit for some time now, I really didn't want to disappoint her and tell her that I really didn't feel like going. This was my very last day before starting my chemo treatments. I was so preoccupied with depression before the *BIG DAY!* After having such a wonderful morning at my hairdresser's, how could I fall into this depression?! The depression consumed me like never before, and I couldn't stand seeing Brittanie's smiling face disappointed. How could I say no, and tell her I couldn't go. So we rested up a little after she came home from school and Paul and I went ahead for the visit. Brittanie chose to drive and acted as our personal chauffeur. She was so excited and talkative the entire trip.
I just sat in the back seat going deeper and deeper into my depression. When we drove up on the campus of the TV 5 Studios, I experienced a sudden

spirit of elation as though someone breathed a breath of energy into my body. The campus was simply beautiful and so well manicured. We were so very impressed. As Brittanie parked her car and we walked onto the grounds, one could not be more overwhelmed by the towers of technology that it took to house and maintain such an industry. There were satellites, cameras, and security everywhere.

She walked us into the studio with her badge in hand just like a little girl on her first day of school! Just as we walk in (approximately 4:50 p.m.) It was time for the 5:00 News. We immediately saw two of my favorite reporters of all...Rob Martin, the infamous chief weather meteorologist, and the 5:00 News Anchor herself, Cynthia Tyler! He was very handsome and she was beautiful. The cameras just didn't do them justice and I made sure I told them!(smile) They both were flattered but had to touch up their make up and run on set to air the 5:00 News. Breaking news was happening all that afternoon. We happened to visit on a huge news day. The local and state election returns were going on, along with fires, plane crashes and you name it. I was just so glad to meet them and feel their kindness even in the midst of their schedules. They were so sweet and personable.

Brittanie let us watch Paul Harding, Cynthia Tyler and Rob Martin on set for the 5:00 News. After that we toured the Control Room. We met Warren Farmer, the Executive Producer in the Control Room. Even in the midst of the hectic news day, he was so kind to us. He pointed to the number of television screens and explained how they were able to capture various news stories happening at once. They were also able to cue each reporter as to when they should report. He further showed us various other news stations airing simultaneously that they also monitored. It seemed all so fascinating and encompassing. She particularly wanted us to meet one of the producers who she'd grown very fond of who she nicknamed *"Sunshine"*. He was a terrific young man who had grown fond of her as well. He was a dear friend who was a mirrored reflection of Brittanie's infectious personality. Brittanie possessed a unique talent of keeping everyone around her happy. Unfortunately, *"Sunshine"* was leaving the station that week and was going back home, which was up North. It was so good to finally meet her buddy. She talked about him often!

We then went to the Newsroom where the heart and soul of the news takes place daily. It was a most intense area. Located also in this room were copier machines that printed scripts in succession that the Interns were responsible for sorting and getting to the Producers and other personnel. This process is done on a timely basis in order to have reports ready for upcoming news slots for the News Anchor Reporters. This was part of Brittanie's job and she demonstrated the process to us. She introduced us to Lauren, one of her friends who was a new kid on the block for TV 5. She was intently preparing scripts for the evening's election returns. She told us that she would have a very long evening at work since it was an election night. She was responsible for ordering food catered for staff that stayed throughout the evening. Of course, Brittanie being the *"always ready to munch lunch kid"*, helped herself to some of the food with no shame; knowing that she was not scheduled to work that evening!! (smile)

We were so pleased to meet a few of the other reporters on staff. We met Bob Weeks, who was new to the city and anchor of the newly launched "News Update" that aired at 11:00 p.m. each evening. I also met Amy Hunt, the Health and Medical Reporter. I reminded her that she'd just completed a report at my company on teen pregnancy in Georgia. She remembered and was so kind to take time to talk with me. I complimented her health reports and told her how we so looked forward to hearing their informative issues. We met Paula Day, who's also one of my favorite reporters. She shared very kind words to us of Brittanie's personality and told us how proud we should be of her accomplishments since she'd been with the station.

Paula promised us that Brittanie had a very promising future in news reporting and would do well wherever she landed. We are very proud of her. Paula became a personal dear friend of mine. She sent e-mails to me nearly every other week, checking up on me and always assuring me she was praying for me. Her kind gestures of concern touched my heart deeply. As busy and hectic as her schedule was at work, she always took time to keep in touch with me. I'll never forget her thoughtful heart.

Our next step was to walk the halls of the studio, where displayed were all of the alumni reporters, events, and history of TV 5. There was a gallery of pictures on the walls throughout the halls that captured legendary moments in TV 5 history. We were so impressed with all the history, and reminisced fondly of reporters and executives of the station who had moved on or who were deceased. It was quite a legacy that made our city proud! We were then on our way out, so as not to disturb anyone else on this very busy news day. Brittanie explained to us that this is the nature of the news industry…everyday is an intense day in producing and delivering the news. Our last step was to view the master control room, where we were only able to peek inside. It was too busy to go in. We could not leave without taking a tour of the "Good Morning Atlanta" set where all the musical guests and celebrity guests staged their performances. It was most fascinating! It was the end of a most exciting day that I would have missed out on if I hadn't accepted Brittanie's invitation. I'm glad that I did accept. We could not stop talking about our visit all the way home. I was so glad that she was able to turn a most depressing day for me into a day of thrilling joy. How wonderful. It too was most memorable!

Tuesday, July 15, 2008- After such an exciting day of the TV 5 Studio tour, we wanted to end the day with a family prayer. We had been planning for some time to designate time when the girls would be at the house to have family prayer time. There was so much to pray for...especially since it was on the eve of my very first chemo treatment. Dana acknowledged each of our prayer requests. Dana was experiencing the fight of her life in her job career. Brittanie was so overwhelmed with school, her Internship, and missing her little Jordynn who was away for the summer with her Dad and his family. Of course I needed continued prayer to sustain me through this cancer fight. Paul needed encouragement just trying to hold the family all together. We really needed a powerful blessing from the Lord for our family.

We ate dinner, had some great moments amongst ourselves, then we all assembled downstairs in our family room for prayer. Dana has become one of our most spiritual prayer warriors in the family with her awesome growth in the Lord, so she chose to lead us in prayer. Before she prayed, she acknowledged prayer requests that we each sought from the Lord. She declared that the Lord will answer all of our prayers. We were already emotionally full and touched by Dana's knowing in the spirit what we all needed from the Lord. It was so beautiful! Amaya even joined us in prayer. She was like a little prayer warrior herself in tune to our every prayer and cry. She prayed right along with us…with cries as only a child could give. Dana began to lead us in prayer as all our cries joined hers. The Lord moved that night in our home in a way we've never seen. His power consumed us all. We all cried, prayed, and received God's choice blessings. Each one of us began to speak confirmations of what the Lord had spoken into our lives for each other. What a moment that was for our family. It was a night to remember. We all left feeling challenged and changed forever!

CHAPTER 16
FIRST OFFICIAL DAY OF CHEMOTHERAPY AND THE PAINFUL SIDE EFFECTS TO FOLLOW

Wednesday, July 16, 2008-Today is officially my first day of chemotherapy. Finally! This first day's treatment was not chemo, but a prerequisite treatment to it, which is named Herceptin. Herceptin is an antibiotic treatment that serves as a blocker of cells that multiply rapidly reproducing more cancer cells. I would have to undergo this treatment every week for 1 year. This treatment, unlike chemotherapy would not be harmful to my good cells causing sickness or hair loss. The use of Herceptin has to be monitored for heart problems that could occur. This monitoring of my heart was done on a quarterly basis as treatment was given. I had to visit the Cardiologist quarterly, where they performed an echocardiogram on my heart.

My very first treatment of the Herceptin lasted only 45-50 minutes. I was given a Tylenol tab along with a Benadryl drip prior to the Herceptin as accompanying medications. I slipped into a peaceful sleep, only to have my first treatment over within an hour. We left the GEORGIA CANCER CENTER only to return the very next day for the first real chemo treatment.

Thursday, July 17, 2008-We returned for my first chemotherapy treatment. I felt anxious about receiving it, but knew this would finally be the beginning of my fight against this dreaded disease. I had so many obstacles to go through to get to this point. So as anxious as I felt, I was glad to start this battle. I went in for the routine visit to the lab for them to check my weight, blood pressure, temp, and draw my blood. Thankfully, they were able to access my port to draw my blood. Hallelujah! It felt so good not to have my arm poked.

I then went in for my visit with Dr. Sharian. He was especially busy as usual, but when he visited with you, he gave you his undivided attention. I liked that. We were able to ask any questions that we had. Paul accompanied me to each and every one of these visits. I don't know what I would have done without my husband! I was eager to get my test results from my MRI biopsy. I was beginning to think that Dr. Sharian did not have the results yet since I hadn't heard from Dr. Harland. I expected her to be the doctor to call me first with the results since the tests were done at the BREAST CANCER CENTER office. Fortunately, as Dr. Sharian was updating me on all my test results and status of my condition, he said he did have the results of my MRI biopsy. I nervously braced myself. Surprisingly, he was as excited as we were, when he said that it was very good news! He informed me that the test results showed there was no sign whatsoever of cancer in the right breast! I could not contain myself. My tears just flowed. For the first time since learning of my cancer and receiving one report of bad news after another, I finally had some hope and something good to cling to. I could only think, I have one healthy breast...thank

God! I completely tuned out what he said of all the other lab results received. I was just glad that my other breast did not show cancer...THANK YOU LORD!

I then prepared to go in for my chemo treatment. I had no idea what to expect, but could only imagine it would consist of what I'd read in materials given to me via the GEORGIA CANCER CENTER. I must say, from the information I read, the symptoms and side effects after treatment were so overwhelming. I did not look forward to the episodes of sickness that the reading materials predicted. The office was thorough in making sure I had all medications needed to combat the side effects from the treatment. I would receive two forms of chemo treatment today. They consisted of Taxotere and Carboplatin. They both were given by infusion into the vein intraveniously. I received these treatments every 3 weeks. Common side effects of the Taxotere are: low white blood cell count; low red blood cell count; fluid retention; nausea; diarrhea; mouth sores; hair loss; fatigue, weakness; and nail changes.

Common side effects of the Carboplatin are: low blood counts; nausea; taste changes; hair loss;

weakness; burning sensation; abdominal pain; diarrhea; constipation; mouth sores; infection; and cardiovascular problems. Oh my! Please God…help me survive all this poison. The Taxotere was given to me first. This unusual treatment consisted of the nurses putting gloves on my hands and placing my gloved hands in a bucket of ice. This is done because the Taxotere is such a strong treatment and can cause your fingernails to come off and discolor. Placing the gloved hands in a bucket of ice protects the nails and hands from harm. It's a freezing cold process, but must be done. I completed that particular treatment, and boy was I glad that was over. The next chemo treatment I was given was the Carboplatin. I don't remember which of these treatments was stronger. I was finally done with my very first chemo treatment session. The total time to undergo both was 3 hours. I was feeling very weak. Paul and I left the office with me feeling pretty woozy…but glad to go home.

I stayed home all that night bracing myself for whatever reactions I would have to the treatment. Even though I'd read what the side effects to the treatments would be, I had no idea how soon I would become effected. I was forewarned by the nurses, that everyone does not react the same to the medications. I must admit that I was pretty nervous about it all. Surprisingly enough, I waited until 12:00 midnight and didn't see or feel any drastic reactions...I was so glad.

Friday, July 18, 2008-I had to go back to GEORGIA CANCER CENTER for a shot of Neulasta.
This is a *"killer"* (as I called it) shot. This shot serves as a white blood cell booster. It is a medication, injected as a shot in the arm (it can also be shot in the abdomen) that help your body make more of its own natural white blood cells to help protect you against chemotherapy related infection. A low white blood cell count or an infection can place the administering of your chemotherapy treatment on hold. I will be receiving this injection the next day after each chemo treatment. I really dreaded this shot. The shot is injected in the back of the arm or in the stomach. Of course I always received mine in the back of my arm. There is no immediate pain in receiving the shot, but

you must take Tylenol or some kind of acetaminophen afterward to help block the pain. The pain that follows later can be unbearable!

On this same day, I had a follow up appointment with Dr. Norman Foster, the Surgeon who performed the surgery to place my port in my chest. By this time, I was healing quite well from the surgery. I simply had to go in for Dr. Foster to check the incision. It was a quick in and out visit. Dr. Foster only said that I would need to come back to have the port removed once my chemo treatment was completed. I was glad to leave and make it home before the affects of my Neulasta shot would take effect.

Hours later, the pain from the Neulasta shot started along with more pain the next day from the chemotherapy. The pain became more than I could bear. At approximately 4:00 p.m. into the evening, I began to experience the full effects of the havoc these medications bring upon the body. My legs, back, arms, and chest began to hurt like I'd never experienced in my life! I remember hurting so bad in my chest that it felt like my chest cavity was separating itself from my chest wall. It really felt like my heart was coming out of my body. I've never experienced a heart attack before nor knew what it felt like, but I could only imagine that a heart attack felt like this. I literally could not breathe nor relieve myself of this pain. I began to call the nurses on call from GEORGIA CANCER CENTER.

Paul was on his way home from his daughter Janise's home after visiting our grandchildren, Zebria and Zoe. I didn't want to alarm him or Brittanie anymore than necessary, but I had to find out if this pain was normal. When I left GEORGIA CANCER CENTER Thursday afternoon after my chemo treatments, they asked me to report anything out of the ordinary...and trust me, this was clearly an extraordinary pain. My God, what was happening to me?! I remember a very kind nurse calling me back moments after I left a message at the GEORGIA CANCER CENTER. He began to tell me that I was experiencing a normal reaction to the Neulasta. What was happening to me, was that my bone marrow was breaking down while the Neulasta was making more neutrophils (or white blood cells). I could feel every single bone marrow breaking and separating in my body. How painful! I could only describe it as what I'd imagine *"napalm"* would feel like exploding in my bones! Every tissue, joint, and bone in my body felt like it was tearing itself away from my body. My God, please let me live through this night!

The level of pain medication given me had to be increased. I finally took sleep medication to try and help me sleep through the night. Lord, just let me sleep through this night! I need you Lord, I prayed, more than ever! I believe he heard me...I drifted off to sleep...only to experience more pain the next day with nausea and diarrhea to follow. I could only pray that days from this day...I would feel some relief. The first week of chemo was an experience I will never forget!

CHAPTER 17

OH NO...

THERE GOES MY HAIR!

Week of July 24, 2008-All this week, I remember feeling afraid to comb my hair. All I could think of was clumps of my hair coming out, and emotionally, I was not ready to see that! I could only imagine my going bald with no hair to speak of. As much as you expect this kind of thing to happen during this journey...the sight of it can be somewhat overwhelming. I think it was harder on Paul and the girls to watch me lose my hair. All I could remember was one of Paul's ex coworkers, Angie, telling me that you will lose your hair exactly 10-14 days after your first chemo treatment. I had my first treatment 7/17/08...so I assumed I would start losing strands by 7/27. How nervous and anxious I made myself...when I should have focused on feeling better.

I remember the pain, cramping, nausea, diarrhea, and vomiting ending during this week. It seemed that I was sick for exactly a week. Thursday, July 24, 2008 was probably my first day of feeling completely free from any illness. I still remember lingering feelings of sickness, as much as I wanted to rid myself of it. Nevertheless, I began to celebrate each day of health. I would send my e-mail updates out to my church family, my biological family, and my co-workers. I would tell them about my first week surviving chemo and how I was feeling at the time. With the pain I'd been experiencing for the past week from chemo, the ability to send and receive e-mails and talk to folks on the phone was quite a feat.

Each week following chemo treatment, I had to have my labs monitored to check the status of my white blood cell counts, platelets and other indicators. If my white blood count was low, I could not go out or interact with others. My visits from guests at my home were eliminated as well. I was also restricted from eating salads if my counts were low. Well, you could have just locked me up in a room and thrown away the key! I love salad and would feel deprived if I couldn't eat it. But I had to ward off any foods that might transfer germs of any kind...and salad and open food bars were prime examples. I did whatever I needed to do to take proper precautions and stay healthy. I would eat my salad when my cell counts were normal. I could not wait! (smile)

Wednesday July 30, 2008-This day I had to have another treatment for Herceptin. Thank God Herceptin is not a form of chemo, only an antibiotic. My labs yielded a great report! My counts were good and I could go out around people and receive visitors without concern of my immune system being compromised. Even though, my visits were limited, I was thrilled that I could go to church. Staying away from my church family was a real challenge throughout this journey. I really loved and missed them. My family was able to visit me; that made my isolation time tolerable.

Friday, August 1, 2008-My hair began to come out in strands...right on schedule. It was an uncontrollable loss. I could not stop, or slow the process of the hair loss. The strands came out with each combing of my hair, and sometimes just to the touch. I began collecting my hair strands and putting them in a zip lock bag. It was hard to endure.

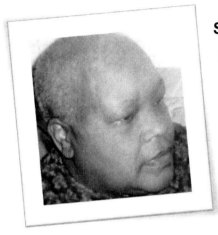

Saturday, August 2, 2008-My hair is now coming out in huge clumps daily. Days after this, it began to come out from the root. With so much loss, Paul, at my request, began to cut my hair with scissors to a very low level. This made the loss of the rest of my hair less painful. My God, I thought, it is really happening! My zip lock bag of hair grew with each combing and touch of my hair. By now my bag was full of hair. The loss of hair on a woman's head is always hard. Our hair is our glory. I was very emotional about losing my hair, not only because of the pride of my appearance as a woman, but also because my hairdresser had just restored my hair to its ultimate health and radiance. I received compliments wherever I went.

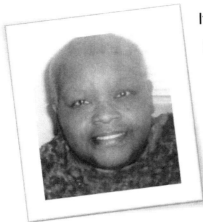 It was bouncy, shiny and beautiful. Oh my, how I prayed to the Lord for a healthy replacement of my hair, once my chemo treatments were all over. I desired for my hair to be as beautiful as before! After many tears and much heartbreak, the Lord gave me a feeling of consolation that the loss of hair is temporal, but the loss of life is permanent. He had given me another chance at life...I was going to live, so why complain about something as minor as hair. It was such a calming revelation for me. My anxieties and fears were at peace!

CHAPTER 18

FIRST SUNDAY BACK TO CHURCH AFTER 3 MONTHS

Sunday, August 3, 2008-Well this is a very important day in my life. It's my first Sunday back to church services since I left prior to my illness on June 22, 2008. It was an experience that seemed surreal. All I did, for a little over a month while I was away from church, was dream of getting back to experiencing the presence of God in the fellowship of his people. I really missed the ministry.

My church has the most powerful move of God ever! It is the most spiritual fulfillment one would want. The Lord's presence is felt in song, the preaching of the word, prayer, testimony, and fellowship.

I had to enter the church via the balcony area because I was unable to be exposed to crowds of people. There in the balcony, I was able to interact with the service with very limited contact with people. Even though I was so glad to be in the presence of the spirit, I really wanted to hug and kiss the members to let them know how much I'd missed them. The Praise and Worship ministry was so anointed. How I enjoyed hearing and feeling the presence of the Lord through song, and His Word. My communion with the Lord allowed me to reminisce on my experience with this cancer thus far. I replayed in my mind, my painful visits to the doctors' offices, taking the chemo treatments, and the roller coaster ride that the Lord had allowed me to experience. I never questioned why the Lord allowed this extraordinary journey to come upon me I just wanted Him to get me through it. The worship songs and music penetrated my very being. I became lost in God's presence and one with His spirit. It was one of the most amazing experiences I've had in a very long time.

While enjoying my visit back at my church, much was revealed to me spiritually. This detour in my life had caused a much closer walk with the Lord than I'd ever had before. I perceived my life so differently. I heard the voice of the Lord more audibly, and felt his presence more powerful than I ever thought imaginable. It seemed that I was the only person in the room with the Lord along with His incense filled aroma. My family sat next to me each Sunday in the balcony. They could only watch me cry uncontrollable tears. They could not even imagine what I was feeling. My Pastors' words spoke right to my heart and were more poignant than ever. The Lord prepared a message each Sunday I came, just for me! We would make our exit quickly near the end of services so as not to come in contact with people. It was hard not to come in contact with them, and then once I did, it was very hard not to be able to hug them and greet them in love. Nevertheless, I was glad to be able to get back to church…and the Lord's spirit met me there every time!

Sunday, August 3, 2008-August 3rd was also my parents' 62nd wedding anniversary. I could not wait to get home to call them, congratulate them, and tell them about my day in church. When I arrived home, we received the sad news that my neighbor's son, Thomas, who grew up in the neighborhood as a very little boy, was killed in a tragic car accident that morning around 3:00 a.m. As wonderful a day as I was having, my heart was saddened by this news. Thomas had just graduated the day before from West Georgia College, and I remember peering out my window watching him celebrate with his family and friends in his front yard. He playfully ran in the street with his graduation cap and gown on. He was never so proud and excited! How tragic for his family and for mine. My girls grew up with him from little children. We all went over to visit with his Mom and family and offered our condolences.

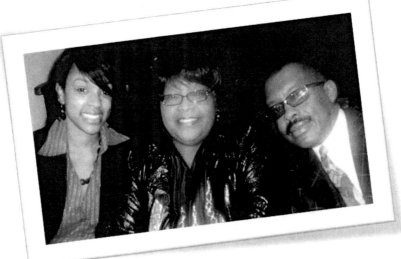

Again, the Lord spoke in every experience in my life. Thomas's death spoke clearly to me of life and how short it is. We must make every single day of our lives count and never take it for granted. How young he was with his dreams and future ending in an instant fatal car accident. One of his best girlfriends from school was in the car with him and was ultimately killed as well.

I spent the afternoon pondering his memories and prayed a special prayer for his family and friends.

CHAPTER 19
GOODBYE MRS. SANDERS

Wednesday, August 6, 2008- I met a wonderful lady by the name of Mrs. Sanders. I remember seeing her walking through the chemo lab with her husband days earlier for the tour that they would take new patients on to show them the facility and what they would have to go through. I fondly remembered my own tour and imagined the fear she must have felt. I learned that Mrs. Sanders had colon cancer. The worse part of her cancer is that she had a tumor on an area of her colon that made it inoperable. When I saw her, it struck me that she was a very attractive woman with beautiful long hair. Her locks were curled so nice each time she would come. Later she began to wear scarves.

The chemo had taken its' toll on her beautiful locks, as it did us all. Mrs. Sanders had a 13 year old young daughter who would accompany her and her husband to the office. I remember her daughter having the saddest look on her face. No doubt, the suffering of her Mom had quite an effect on her as well.

One thing that impressed me about Mrs. Sanders was that she really loved the Lord, and each time she would come into the office for treatment, she would always talk, full of zeal, about how she knew the Lord was going to heal her. Her faith was really amazing. No matter how she was feeling, or how weak she became, she continued to declare how the Lord was her healer...just keep the faith.
I remember seeing her strength weaken and her body noticeably diminishing. I remember missing her coming into the office for nearly a week or more. When I finally saw her again, she told me that she'd been very sick and was hospitalized for a week and a half. Mrs. Sanders told me that her cancer was a rare case and the chemo was not effective for her. It was just not doing her any good at all! Paul immediately got up and abruptly ran out of the waiting room in tears upon hearing Mrs. Sanders's words. He found it extremely painful to hear that the chemo was not

helping her! It was more than he could take. Paul lost his Mom to breast cancer many years ago...the painful thought of her death, and the thought after all these years that chemo would not be able to help someone, was unbearable for him to hear. It was visibly emotionally painful for him.

Mrs. Sanders was aggravated with having to continually come for treatment and it was not helping her.
The chemo was having no positive effect on her cancer. The doctors, however, insisted on continually treating her. Apparently, it was their opinion that it was more beneficial to treat her than not. I totally trusted Dr. Sharian and his professional opinion. I could only pray that the Lord would send her a miracle.

I remember the last time I saw her at the office. She slowly walked in, now needing assistance from her husband to walk. She caught my eye as I was sitting waiting for my labs and treatment, and she gave me the biggest smile. She sat next to me and could only lay her head on my shoulder. She told me how bad and weak she felt. I comforted her, prayed with her and told her she was in good hands. I told her the Lord would take care of her and ease her pain. That moment pained me, but it was a conversation that was etched in my mind. No matter what happened, she never waivered in her faith that God was going to heal her and her illness was in his hands.

When I came into the office for one of my treatments, I missed seeing her and asked the lab nurse where was she. I was saddened to learn that Mrs. Sanders died on Sunday, October 5th. How my heart broke...I wished I could have told her goodbye. Each patient was very special to the staff. When they lose a patient, they would send a card to the family signed by the entire staff. I learned that her wake and funeral would be held on the following Friday and Saturday evenings. We really wanted to attend. Since I'd just had my treatment, I was much too weak to go. We'd made plans to go to the wake. Ultimately, Paul stayed home to be with me. I could only think of her 13 year old daughter and how distressed she must have been to lose her Mom so young. My daughter, Brittanie tried calling her daughter to show her love and support. Brittanie too was suffering with her Mom with cancer. She wanted to share words of love to comfort her. Paul called Mr. Sanders's home and spoke with her husband's brother. The family was having a difficult time with her loss. Paul gave him comforting words and assured him that we were praying for the family.

I never forgot Mrs. Sanders's words, or her phenomenal faith. I do believe that her prayers were answered. The Lord healed her and took her on to be with Him. That is the greatest healing of all. She would no longer have to suffer the pain and agony of her illness anymore. What a remarkable woman! I will never forget her strength, tenacity, and spirit!

CHAPTER 20
TREATMENT HALFWAY MARK-AND "IT'S BRITTANIE'S BIRTHDAY"!

Tuesday, September 9, 2008-I had an appointment today with Dr. Harland, my breast Surgeon at the BREAST CANCER CENTER office. This is the halfway point of my chemo treatment (the 3rd of 6 treatments), and she needed to examine me via ultrasound to see how the chemo was effecting the tumor in my breast. Dr. Harland reviewed my x-rays from the ultrasound and had great news for me when Paul and I went into the office to see her. My tumor mass was ¾ smaller than the original size! The smaller tumors were all gone as well. She was so excited, but not nearly as excited as Paul and I were!

We were thrilled beyond measure to hear this news. The chemo was doing the job that it was designed to do. I began to praise God for His hand in this portion of my journey. It is because of Him we are healed and progress as successfully as we do in any illness. I am a firm believer in medicine, but it is our faith in God and his powerful hand that causes the medicine to work as it should. I thank God to have Him in my life!

Dr. Harland then had me go to the scheduling department to get set up for surgery for my bilateral mastectomy. Dr. Harland was glad that both Paul and I decided to have the bilateral surgery. We didn't want to endure the pain of having one breast removed and the cancer recurring in my other breast. I did not want to experience this pain again years down the road. Ultimately, Paul and I were at peace with the decision of having both breasts removed. I also had scheduled surgery with Dr. Debra Lindsey, my Plastic Surgeon for my reconstruction procedure. The date was set! My surgery was scheduled for December 16, 2008. It was important that I kept the date of December 11th free for my daughter, Brittanie's graduation from college. So this date was perfect! This might sound hard to believe, but I was actually excited about surgery! I knew this would mark a point in my journey of Phase II and I would be all done with chemotherapy. Anything would be better than having to undergo the brutal experience of chemotherapy. I thought...nothing could be worse!

Wednesday, September 10, 2008-My appointment for Consultation with Dr. Lindsey, my Plastic Surgeon was scheduled today. Dr. Lindsey's consultation consisted only of her looking at my breasts and determining what type reconstruction surgery she would perform. She laughed and humorously said that my breasts would be lifted and perkier than ever...I concurred and chuckled... "let's do this!" (smile)

Wednesday, September 17, 2008-I met an incredible young lady at the cancer office by the name of Monica Harris. Monica was suffering from cancer of her stomach. She'd already undergone several tests as a result of experiencing severe pain in her stomach. She was later diagnosed with cancer. I met Monica in the chemo lab where we had our treatments. Right away, we talked for seemingly hours. We'd become instant (BF's...best friends...smile) Since I'd been undergoing treatment longer than Monica, I would take time and familiarize her with all the services and benefits available to patients with cancer. She was amazed by all the assistance available via the American Cancer Society and other cancer agencies. We would collect books, magazines, journals, wigs, and hats that the office had available along with information educating us on cancer. It was so much fun. We would try on wigs and hats and critique one another on what looked good on us, and which ones we needed to leave on the rack!(smile) We would sit in our chair taking our treatments and talk about our cancer, our pains, life, and how the cancer had affected our lives. Monica loved the Lord as I did, so we talked a lot about the Lord and our spiritual experiences with him. She and her family were great believers in the use of natural herbs, fruits, vegetables, and juice drinks for the cure of cancer. They vowed to help her homeopathically to prevent the continued use of chemo. Ultimately, she chose to go ahead with the administration of chemotherapy to save her life. I knew she would make such an impact on my life.

We had so much fun together, and if she got to the office for her treatment before me, she would reserve a chair right next to her for me. We were like childhood school girls all over again! Our talks and friendship made our sufferings less painful and stressful. What an amazing friend!

Monday, September 29, 2008-My tumor markers were too high at this point in my treatment, and Dr. Sharian became concerned. A tumor marker is a substance found in the blood, urine, or body tissues that can be elevated in cancer. When I started my treatment, my markers were 55. At this point in my treatment, it was about 48…it should have been in the range of 35-45. I became so upset! Please Lord don't let anything go wrong now. Even though my tumors had decreased its size substantially, my markers were still too high.

I immediately did the only thing I knew to do when I knew I needed a miracle from the Lord. I contacted my Pastors and Caregroup Leader Sisters and asked them to pray for me. Caregroup Leaders at my church consists of 13 women who are in leadership positions over the congregation of women. Each of them are prayer warriors in their own right. I knew they would pray for me with such power that I would receive the miracle that I needed from the Lord.

In order to test the status of my tumor markers, I had to once again undergo a PET scan. I'd already had one of these tests, so I knew what to expect. I went to Epicure, the PET and CT scan office across the street from the Georgia Cancer Center. I had to fast hours before the scan to allow the test to show what they needed to see without excessive food in my system. I received my injection intravenously to insert the dye needed to assist them in administering this test. Unfortunately, they were not allowed to access my port to inject the dye. The PET scan took approximately 45 minutes. Since this in an open enclosure machine, I was not as terrified as I was with the MRI. Once the test was completed, I was able to be on my way, get something to eat (I was starved) and await the test results from my doctor's office.

My next visit to the doctor was filled with great news. My test results from the PET scan for my tumor markers and labs were good. My tumor markers were at 42, and I could not have been more thrilled! My Caregroup Leaders at church were so happy, but not surprised. They all knew the power of prayer, and they prayed expecting great results. I was so relieved!

Monday, October 13, 2008- This is Brittanie's 24th birthday and I am saddened that I have to be in bed sick on her birthday. I informed both she and Dana that I would not be able to celebrate their birthdays this year, due to my illness, but I promised to more than make up in celebrations next year when I'm well. Not to worry, she and her friends hosted a series of birthday celebration events planned for her. She had a week long list of activities planned starting with the weekend... Friday, October 10, 2008. She enjoyed herself so much, that by the time she got to her birthday on the 13th, I think she was exhausted from all the festivities!(smile)

Tuesday, October 14, 2008-I was experiencing severe headache pain on a daily basis. I thought, Lord I am undergoing enough pain with the chemotherapy I didn't need any added stress.

I reported this pain to Dr. Sharian after suffering with the headaches for a period of time. He then ordered a CT scan for me to make sure there was nothing more severe going on with my head other than stress. The cancer office has the facility onsite to administer this test, so I had it done on this date. The CT scan only takes about 20-25 minutes. This simple test consisted of an injection of dye intravenously. Days later, Dr. Sharian gave me the good news that the test did not show anything medically wrong. All was well. It appeared that I was experiencing extreme stress as a result of the treatments. I was able to take the same pain medications I took for the chemo for my headaches. The headaches subsided days after my CT scan.

CHAPTER 21

LAST DAY OF CHEMOTHERAPY TREATMENT!

Wednesday, October 29, 2008-This was a day I will never forget! It was the last day of my chemotherapy treatment! YAY! I had long awaited this day. With each treatment, the nurses and I would count down….3 more treatments…2 more treatments…1 more treatment! I could not wait for this dreaded pain to end. I was all smiles the entire day. It was even more special, because not only was my husband with me, but my daughter, Brittanie was able to come as well. She went into work and they let her go home early so she could join me. How happy I was! She had always talked of wanting to accompany me for my treatments for support.

I was able to introduce all of the staff to Brit. They were delighted to meet her. They shared with her what a great patient I was, and she told them how highly I spoke of them as well. She sat in a treatment chair next to me and saw what I experienced every 3 weeks. Brittanie had me dying laughing at what she did. She not only ate all my snacks that I normally brought to each treatment, but she ate up many of the snacks that were designated ONLY for the patients! She then fell asleep in the treatment chair that she was occupying which was also designated only for the patients. Thank goodness this was a slow day for patients. I thought to myself, how shameless she was, but I enjoyed every moment of having her there with me! (smile)

It is a tradition with the office when a patient completes their treatment sessions of chemo, to host a party for them. At this party, all of the staff attended, they would throw confetti at you, give you a certificate of completion, and shower you with many hugs and kisses. I added the tears of joy! No one understands like the patient, how it feels to complete this part of the journey. It is a joy and relief! Monica was there at the office this day and she celebrated with me! She awaited her last day as well….which would be soon.

I remember taking a moment and fondly remembering Mrs. Sanders. How I wish she could have been there to celebrate with me. How I wished that she could have made it through the end of her treatments…and lived! I know the joy she was experiencing in heaven, was by far greater than anything I could have enjoyed. But how I missed her! I could feel her spirit smiling at me with that beautiful smile that only she could give. It was a wonderful day for me and my family. I could now look forward to the next phase of my treatment, the surgery. Who wanted to think of surgery…I just wanted to finish enjoying the party! What a day I had!

Friday, October 31, 2008-I had to go and have an echo cardio exam at Fairway Fayette Hospital, at the Crowne Point location. The hospital was just up the street from the GEORGIA CANCER CENTER. It is the policy of the office that you have your heart examined quarterly when you are undergoing the treatment of Herceptin. This treatment can be very harsh on the heart. My test results came back very good. My heart was in great shape and had not undergone any adverse affects from the Herceptin. My celebration of the end of chemotherapy treatment continued!

CHAPTER 22
GENERAL ELECTION DAY 2008

Tuesday, November 4, 2008-IT'S GENERAL ELECTION DAY 2008! What can I say about today! Since my diagnosis and my leave from work, June 30, 2008, I laid in bed struggling with my illness. I also had time to attentively watch the Presidential campaign, the candidates, their platforms, debates, and news analysts' views on the election. I must say, it was the most invigorating part of my illness. Even though, mentally, I was experiencing the fight of my life with my emotions, the campaign proved quite enlightening for me! I learned so much about politics, the science of campaigning, and the results of effective politics. The career of a politician can be one of the most self-serving professions I know. Everyone does what they have to do to promote themselves and their interests. Even though Politics is a profession where one vows to serve the public and place the needs of the people first, one tries to achieve their goals at all cost. The highest office in government becomes the ultimate goal. Ironically, I eventually grew to respect governmental officials, as I would see them debate their opponents passionately. Candidates debate with spirited exchanges, only to find at the end of the debates, they were like compassionate friends who not only really respected one another, but vowed to promote the unified interests of the country. Their passion accompanied with attacking, words would quickly turn into pats on the back, and compliments of one another for a job well done! I found it simply amazing!

The news commentators and hosts were just as phenomenal as the politicians. I would watch them debate one another with such intensity. At the end of each session, they would end their debates with much respect and camaraderie. How amazing! I was already a devoted fan of news and spent hours watching all the cable network news shows, even before my illness. Now I had the time to consistently watch them with great interest in the progress of the campaign. I had a favorite cable news show, which will remain anonymous at this time! (smile)

Due to the weakness in my legs, I knew I could not stand in a long line for early voting. So I simply had Paul go to the polling spot and pick up an absentee ballot for me. I filled it out quickly and mailed it right back in. I felt as proud completing that ballot and mailing it in, as if I'd stood in line for 5-6 hours along with all the other voters. Brittanie stood in line for 6 hours. She was determined to stay in line until her vote was cast regardless of the agonizing wait. It was by far, the most amazingly charged, historical, and refreshing campaign ever!

Wednesday, November 5, 2008-I was as excited about this day as ever! I was like a little kid on Christmas Eve, running around with the expectancy of receiving bundles of gifts. I wanted to prepare snacks for the election returns that night after 7:00 p.m. and stay up to the bitter end to watch and be a part of history. It was reminiscent of Super Bowl Sunday...when I would stop by the store and purchase snacks and soft drinks to enjoy the game! I wanted to take a nap early that day, so I could be all rested and ready to stay up as late as needed to enjoy the election results.

I'd just had my last chemo treatment October 29th, and wasn't feeling the best the night of the election returns, but I was determined to stay up and watch this historical night of events. I wanted nothing more than to witness this occasion first hand. I was feeling fine all day that day, but then at approximately 6:00 p.m. or 7:00 p.m. that evening, I began feeling pain in my bones like never before. I began to pray, "dear God, please don't let me be sick, please don't let me be sick…not now!" I could feel myself declining by the minute and could not stand the pain any longer. The pain meds that I took for the chemo rendered me immobile. As a result, I was out like a light. So there I went, dozing off to sleep on this most exciting night!

I remember early evening election results, and hearing Barack Obama win much of the Northeast states. When I heard that he'd won Pennsylvania, Virginia, Illinois and Michigan…I knew he was on his way, and it would be one of the most exciting elections ever! However, I was drifting off into

another world, a world where I would not get to enjoy the moment. I was gone. I slept through the most informative commentary imaginable by the news pundits I had grown to love. I remember my phone ringing at approximately 10:30 p.m. or 10:45 p.m. that evening. It was my daughter Brittanie. She was so excited that she could barely talk! I could hear the roar of voices in the background of people celebrating and partying or whatever they were doing! It was all so unclear. She shouted…. "MOMMY, Barack Obama is President of the United States!" I hung up quickly, feeling somewhat thrilled and disappointed…all at the same time. The phone rang again. It was my other daughter Dana.
She yelled the same thing… "MOMMY, Barack Obama has won as President of the United States!" All I could hear was her voice seemingly hyperventilating and the cheers of the crowds in the background! A part of my soul began to feel left out. One of the most exciting days of United States history, and I slept through it…oh my God, how could this happen! I felt that I had just awaken from a horrible dream. How could I have missed this all important moment! The returns were happening, and

I was not a part of it. The crowds were cheering on every news network and I laid in bed in pain, in and out of a fog that I could not awaken from.

While the television was on in my room all night, I began to try and focus my eyes on what was happening. My girls were right...every major cable network news station aired the announcement that BARACK OBAMA had been elected as the 44th President of the United States! It was flashing everywhere like neon signs. All I could do was cry continuously. More than the exhilaration of Obama winning the office, in the midst of my medicated state, I heard that he had won the state of Florida! That is my home state, and my dad and I had debated back and forth the entire campaign that Florida would never be a state won by the Democrats. Florida had for years been a Republican state, and would remain in the minds of most. When I heard this news that the Democrats had won Florida and I could see the state blue on screen...I cried harder than ever! It was truly a turning point in Florida politics forever. Barack Obama's win of Florida suddenly awakened me out of sedation! I no longer felt the lethargic effects of my medications. It was truly amazing! This man had come on the scene and revolutionized the world and now, these United States of America. What a phenomena he was!

I lay in bed more alert. I began to think of Mr. Obama's deceased Grandmother. I was saddened by her death, but knowing the Lord and His timing, He knew that He allowed her to go in "His time", and not the time of the election. I viewed her death, on the day before the election, as God's way of allowing her to oversee Barack's life and give him the final seal of approval. It was as though she was telling him to "go ahead…remember all I've taught you, you will be just fine!" My tears continued to flow. My tears were of elation mixed with sadness. I could only lay there in bed after I'd awaken completely from the medications, and watch the aftermath of the returns. I wish I felt well enough to run out into my street and yell at the top of my lungs or shoot fireworks! How proud I was of this moment… how surreal! What an achievement. WHAT AN HONOR!

Thursday, November 6, 2008- I spent this day, again in bed, but feeling more energized and celebrant of the excitement of our nation's win! I decided to make myself feel better, in spite of my pain. So I chose this day to celebrate Barack's win and make up for all the excitement I missed. I caught up on the election news and results that I'd missed the night before. It was an electrifying night! Everyone interviewed had well wishes for our new President elect. All in all, I reconciled in my mind that I was going to be a part of this win in spirit, even if I was unable to enjoy the thrill of the night. It was all so fascinating!

CHAPTER 23

PREPARING FOR BILATERAL MASTECTOMY SURGERY- "JORDYNN HAS A BIRTHDAY"!

Friday, November 14, 2008-I have another consultation with Dr. Harland today. This consultation is in preparation for my surgery scheduled for December 16, 2008. Dr. Harland gave me a final examination, Paul then was escorted to Dr. Harland's office to join me. We were told what to expect before surgery. She explained the next phase in detail. Phase II would consist of a bilateral mastectomy, and the insertion of breast tissue expanders by Dr.

Lindsey. Breast tissue expanders are inserted into the breast cavity along with ports that are inserted as well.

The ports are a source of access for a needle to go in and inject saline fluid to inflate the breast at some point. Phase 3 will be the administration of radiation. I was so not looking forward to radiation, but this will be a "piece of cake" compared to chemotherapy. I'm told that I would experience a burning sensation closer to the end of the radiation treatment along with a sense of fatigue. I was accustomed to extreme fatigue with chemotherapy, so this will be a manageable side effect. Phase 4 would be the actual reconstruction surgery with the insertion of implants. This procedure would take place in approximately 9 months to 1 year after my radiation treatment if not before. Dr. Harland explained the type incision that would be made into the breast for the bilateral mastectomy, and the role that Dr. Lindsey would play in performing plastic surgery immediately following the breast surgery.

Dr. Harland then escorted me to Belinda, the Scheduling Administrator, and she scheduled me for a consultation appointment with Dr. Lindsey, prior to surgery. Belinda also had consent forms for me to sign. She told me she would call me with a list of appointment times and dates for pre-surgery tests, phone appointments, and final procedures. I would certainly have a very busy December coming!

Wednesday, November 19, 2008-I had my last Herceptin treatment appointment before surgery scheduled at GEORGIA CANCER CENTER. I was so happy that this appointment did not include chemotherapy. It made for a lighthearted day without the expectancy of pain in my bones and joints! The Herceptin would continue into the New Year. This was my last treatment of it for 2008. The lab technicians were concerned about a cough and cold that I was getting. They suggested that I get a flu shot, something that I had never had all my life. I have never believed in flu shots and had heard so many negative side effects from it. The idea of being ordered to get one for my own good was beyond my control. I was advised that due to the potentially low level of one's immune system, all patients are required to take it. Our systems can be compromised with the contraction of any kind of colds or flu's. I was further advised that contracting a flu virus could be quite detrimental...and can even cause one to be hospitalized when the patient is going through post chemotherapy treatment. I didn't want to take a chance on being more ill than I'd already been, so I allowed them to give me the shot. Once I completed my Herceptin treatment, they immediately gave me the flu shot. Oh my goodness, I thought, I'm going to be so sick!

I asked the nurse how soon will I feel the effects of the shot? She said it can be as soon as this afternoon, tomorrow, or this week. She asked that I simply take cold medications as I normally would for a cold. I left the office knowing that it was imperative for me to take something right away for colds, to prevent any oncoming illness. I wished everyone a Happy Thanksgiving, Merry Christmas, and Happy New Year since I would not be seeing them again until January 2009.

Monday, November 24, 2008-Jordynn celebrates her 2nd birthday! What a big girl she had become! Grand mommy could not be prouder of her. She is such a receptive, bright little girl, with verbal expressions she'll say at 2 years old that would melt your heart. We normally host a big party for the grand's birthday, but due to my health, we chose to let her celebrate with her father and Grandparents in North Carolina when she visited them in a few weeks. Her Godmothers took her out with their family to a nice restaurant and gave her a life size stuffed Minnie Mouse doll. Only one problem, Jordynn was so scared of the doll that she never even touched her! We thought it was so hilarious. She will grow to love her later. In the meantime, we vowed to host a large party for her 3rd birthday when I was well. I was so grateful to have her in my life…what a joy she is!

CHAPTER 24

"THANKSGIVING DAY"

Thursday, November 27, 2008-Thanksgiving day proved to be a day full of family fun. My family and I normally spend a long weekend with my parents in Florida for the Thanksgiving holiday, but due to my uncertain health, we chose to stay here in the city of Atlanta. My extended family consists of nearly 40-50 members this includes my parents, my siblings/in-laws, nieces, nephews, grands, and great grands. We so look forward to being altogether once a year. When we don't gather together for this occasion, it really leaves a sad hole in my heart. However, this year, many of our family members were unable to travel to my parents in Florida for the holiday. Nevertheless, I was able to enjoy the day with my sister, Evelyn and her husband, Ervin and family. Paul, Dana, Amaya and myself all went to enjoy Thanksgiving dinner with my sister. Brittanie and Jordynn traveled to Washington, D.C. to enjoy the day with Jordynn's Dad's family. What a wonderful day. I was glad to have taste buds (after the chemo) to return and I could enjoy dinner! We ate well, had fun, and ended the day with many hugs.

At the end of the day, I began to reminisce about Thanksgiving dinners from the past with ALL of my family gathered together; the games, the fun, the food, and the love. I really missed being with my parents this year. But I knew this Thanksgiving would be like no other. I had so much to be thankful for this year in particular. I began thanking God first of all for my life.

Life is taken for granted so often, that when our lives are threatened, we have a greater appreciation for the hours of the day, days of the week, months of the year, and years that we pray the Lord will give us to share love with one another. I watched my husband survive horrible memories of the war in Viet Nam, and lived to tell about it and take care of me and my family.

I saw my daughters mature to beautiful young women, complete remarkable college studies, and bless me with two lovely grand-daughters who are the most precious gifts from God. I was blessed to have both my parents still alive and doing well, that meant more to me than the teachings they'd taught me all my life. What an adorable pair of examples for my own life!

So this Thanksgiving proved to be a most memorable one. Even though we weren't able to travel to Florida to be with my parents and the extended family, we all celebrated with our own families and cherished the real meaning of thankfulness. It was a breath of blissful delight!

CHAPTER 25

CONSULTATION WITH PLASTIC SURGEON BEFORE MASTECTOMY SURGERY

Wednesday, December 3, 2008- This day I had my second consultation appointment before surgery with my Plastic Surgeon, Dr. Lindsey. I had given my surgery a lot of thought the nights leading up to this appointment, and I'd had a change of heart concerning my reconstruction procedure. Reading the flyer that was given to me by the surgeon's office, I became quite concerned about the insertion of implants, the quality and life of them, as well as unforeseen complications one can develop from the use of implants. I'd decided that if I only have the breasts removed, I would not go through with the implants. I wanted to simply have the bilateral mastectomy and not have reconstruction at all. I made up my mind to go ahead and simply purchase the prosthetic used to enhance my look. The prosthetic would replace my breasts. I was adamant about not having to medically go back later in life and deal with complications from implants. I thought, with the prosthetic, I would not have the headaches, stress, and complications that implants would cause. Paul and I discussed this further in the car on my way to my consultation with Dr. Lindsey, and he too agreed with my decision. When I walked into her office, my mind was made up.

Dr. Lindsey allowed Tammie, her PA, to see me and go over all the details of my surgery. She told me what to expect, and how I needed to prepare myself for the surgery. I expressed my concern of the surgery with Tammie and told her why I'd decided not to go with the implants and reconstruction surgery. Tammie understood my concerns, but began to advise me on the positive benefits of having the implants done. She informed me of the medical advances that have been made with this procedure since the flyer I was reading had been published. She even told me how it is not a surgery that I would be pressured into doing right away. I can have the mastectomy and wait years later to have the reconstruction and implants done. It would be a natural look to enhance my breasts and I would not have to worry about the trouble of putting on a prosthesis each time I had to go out. Tammie took so much quality time with me to convince me to have the reconstructive surgery. Her conversation was quite impressive.

Paul was in the room with me for the consultation, and he too had been convinced that the implants would be a safe way to go with my reconstruction. One thing about Paul, he supported me in whatever decisions I made. He only wanted me to feel comfortable and happy. I really needed a lot of convincing…and I think I was.

Tammie then proceeded to discuss the procedure in detail with me so I knew what to expect. She also gave me a timetable so I'd know how long the surgery, hospital stay, recovery time, along with preparations I had to make before the surgery. She gave me a list of items I had to purchase before the surgery, one of which was an antibacterial soap used the night before and the morning of surgery. She then gave me a list of prescriptions to have filled prior to my surgery.

This would relieve the stress of trying to fill prescriptions after surgery while possibly experiencing pain. Tammie then took me in a room right next to my exam room, where she took pictures of my breasts and chest area only. This is a normal procedure done at the office for all patients before surgery.

I was given a booklet of instructions and a checklist of things to do and not to do prior to surgery. Tammie then directed us to go to another complex of the hospital to have more pre-op, lab work, and x-rays done. I went and had that done and was now able to await the next step in preparation for my surgery.

CHAPTER 26
MY VISIT BACK TO MY JOB BEFORE SURGERY

Thursday, December 4, 2008-I wanted to go back to my job to visit my coworkers after the Thanksgiving holiday and before my surgery on December 16th. Since I was getting my strength back and feeling much better, I decided to go today. It was a particularly perfect day to visit. The weather was not bad, only a mist of rain. I'd really missed seeing everyone and so looked forward to our seeing one another. I'd kept in contact with many of my coworkers, so this would be a great reunion! I had not seen anyone from the office since June 30, 2008. When I arrived in the lobby, I was approached with hugs from the security guard, Anthony. He was a special friend who I would spend hours of time talking to about political, current, and social issues when I was at work. It was especially nice to see him again. Before I even got up to my company's floor, Anthony and I spent a lot of time talking and catching up on my health and what I'd missed discussing with him in the news. We parted vowing to continually keep in touch with one another. I told him that I expected to return to work soon.

When I arrived at my company's floor, I was greeted at the door by EVERYONE! It was such a warm and fun-filled reunion! I had never felt better to see all their faces. Some of the staff were old friends I'd already known. Others were new members who I'd never met before. The new staff proved to be as warm and friendly as the ones I'd worked with for years. What a wonderful visit it was. Everyone complimented me on how well I looked, and to me, the feeling was so mutual. We discussed briefly about my look after losing my hair, but they all adored my stylish new hat! I'd really missed seeing everyone. I then went to the new area of the office where my department had moved…the finance department. The change of atmosphere was so nice and refreshing. I sat and talked for hours with Alyssa, our HR Director, and Cindy, my boss and the Finance Director. We had a wonderful chat and caught up on all we'd missed while I was away.

I then went to visit with many of the other staff members throughout the office and had to wrap my stay up so as not to prolong my time.
I didn't want to overstay my welcome, but really wanted quality time with everyone. We parted with hugs and kisses, and a vow that they would continue to keep me in their prayers. It was a day I won't soon forget. I really felt the sincerity of being missed, how awesome it was!

CHAPTER 27

BRITTANIE GRADUATES AND A MEMORABLE DINNER

Thursday, December 11, 2008-What can I say about this day? It was the graduation of my daughter, Brittanie from Clayton State University. She was graduating from college. We were all so excited! I must take a minute to say something about Brittanie. Brit is my baby girl, and she experienced a lot of obstacles leading up to her big day! She became pregnant her Junior year in college. Like my oldest daughter, Dana, who'd also became pregnant her Junior year in college. I was beginning to believe these girls had lost sight of their careers at this point in their lives, derailing their futures.

My thought was how they could interrupt such an important time in their lives with the expectancy of a child. Didn't they know what a child would mean in their lives while confronting the stress of college?! All the money we'd spent for their education, they both became pregnant before marriage. My whole world suddenly became uncertain. This changed our lives.

One thing I can say about both my girls is that they've always had a strong sense of self and value. They both were not looking at their future and their careers through the same lenses that I was. However, they saw the birth of their daughters as a blessed addition to their own lives, and they would do whatever they had to do to care for them. Nothing thrilled them more. They really embraced their motherly instincts. I knew only one thing; Paul and I would be there for them every step of the way.

They struggled through the morning sickness, the pain of childbirth, and continued their studies in the midst of it all. They both brought two lovely daughters into our lives. They both are simply amazing! How my heart melted with these precious gifts.

Brit's major is Mass Communications and Media Studies. She wants to one day become a local, national, or international news anchor reporter. The summer of 2006 she was given an opportunity to study abroad in Montepulciano, Italy. She would have to raise the funds to go. We went right to work securing the letters needed to mail to family, friends, and church family members to help raise the funds. We were able to secure all the funds necessary in a timely manner for her to go. However, she was approximately 4-6 weeks pregnant.

We talked with her professors, whom initially decided against her going, but then agreed to let her go. In Italy, where she would live and study were steep mountainous terrains. She would have to do strenuous walking and climbing. This would be quite a challenge while pregnant. We would have to secure doctors and hospitals in the area that would be accessible in case of an emergency. This would help provide her with immediate medical care. Brit realized all this before going, but she was determined to make this trip, and attain the knowledge of this once in a life time experience.

We prepared all the necessary documents, deposited the funds she needed to go, and sent her on her way. She was so excited. It was unexplainable. It was hard as a mother to let her go, but all parents want to help support their children accomplish their dreams, especially an extraordinary dream as this one! Her trip and study was an unforgettable experience. She returned home, and had grown tremendously in her pregnancy! Her dad was nearly floored at the airport when he saw her! He was just as concerned about her going away pregnant as I was. Nevertheless, we were so glad to finally have her back home where I could take proper care of her!

Brit had suffered a lot during the last semester of her studies. The summer semester was her last semester before attaining her degree. During the summer she not only had to concentrate on her studies, but she interned at TV 5 News station. In addition to the stress of these classes and internship, was her learning of my cancer. It was very difficult for her to help care for me during this time in her life. Brit remained focused and determined to complete her education...and I encouraged her as much as I could.

So it all came down to this day, December 11th when she would attain her college degree in Mass Communications and Media Studies. To see her march and accept her degree was an emotional one, not only for her, but for me and all of the family. How proud we were of her and her accomplishments. Paul, Dana, Amaya and I were all there to join her in this great achievement. We congratulated her afterward, met many of her professors, classmates and their families, and went on to dinner to celebrate such a great day! Like the day Dana graduated, we couldn't have been more proud of our girls and what they achieved in the midst of their struggles. What we thought would be a problem for them, turned into the greatest opportunity and achievement ever!

Sunday, December 14, 2008-This would once again be my last Sunday at church for awhile. My surgery was scheduled for the following Tuesday, and I wanted to make the best of my last day to fellowship with my church members. I knew I would once again become confined to my home. This entire weekend was a celebration at my church for our Married Couples Conference. This was a weekend of workshops, recreation, and a banquet dinner planned for all married couples. It was very nice. The Sunday banquet dinner after church was a special treat. Little did I know; the marriage conference committee had planned a wonderful surprise for me at the dinner. We all assembled in the ballroom at my church for dinner and the program started. It was such a lovely setting and occasion.

Near the beginning of the program, one of the hosts of the dinner, Melinda Hart, called on Paul to come up. I had no idea what he was called up on stage for. He began to give remarks about my cancer, what I was getting ready to go through this week for my upcoming surgery, as well as the struggles I've had leading up to this point in my life. I sat there in amazement wondering where this was all going. Paul then asked me to come to the stage. V-3, a gospel singing group which consisted of my Pastors' daughters, Latoya, Sacha, and Shelly, gave me the most incredible tribute in song. They have the most angelic voices ever! They have recorded their very first CD...which was an outstanding success! Shelly said words, on behalf of the group, and expressed how they loved and admired me. She further said that they could not even imagine what I was going through, but assured me that they were praying for me that the Lord would see me through this. Her words were so warm and loving...the tears began to flow from my eyes. They then sang a song dedicated to me entitled... *"The Blood that Jesus Shared, Would Never Lose It's Power."* Their voices and harmony were infectiously awesome! Angels from heaven is what they sounded like. So this whole dedication and time was done for me...how awesome is that?!

The rest of the banquet was filled with pictures capturing many of the events held for the married couples all year. Remarks were given by our Pastors. Evangelist Vinson did not let Paul and I leave the dinner without reassuring me with what to expect from the surgery and radiation. She had gone through a similar surgery. She wanted to comfort and prepare me. Evangelist Vinson is an incredible Pastor's wife, Mother, Counselor, and friend.

She always insists on encouraging those she loves. Her words were very comforting and appreciated. I was then able to go into this surgery strengthened in my faith and assured that all was well. The day and dinner was extraordinary, and the love heartfelt!

CHAPTER 28
MORE PRE-SURGICAL TESTS- "DANA CELEBRATES HER BIRTHDAY"!

Monday, December 15, 2008-This is Dana's 29th birthday! She was well aware that I would not be able to celebrate with her for her birthday this year due to my upcoming surgery. She understood and just wanted me to get better. Dana is an incredibly gifted child. She is my first born, and from her early years, she possessed a powerful gift of prayer. Since her days as a child she had the instinctive ability to pray the heart of God. Her prayers were so needed during my illness, and she felt the need to oblige me whenever I needed it. She was also anointed with a singing talent that only the Lord Himself could give.

Though she, like Brittanie, has had her share of disappointments and would lose her way, she's always known how to find her way back to the Lord.

Like Brittanie, Dana had a weekend of birthday celebrations planned with her friends. She had a wonderful time of partying and fun!

This day was also another day of preparation for my surgery. I had an appointment scheduled at the Northwest Women's Center. The purpose of this appointment was to have tests done to help target where my lymph nodes were that had to be removed during my bilateral mastectomy. The technicians at the Women's center had me to dress into a hospital gown and go back to an examination room. In this examination room, the technician administered anesthetics so the doctor could give me a shot in my nipple injecting a certain dye. This needle injection of dye would then enable my breasts to be x-rayed. A male technician was then ordered from another department, and transported me via wheelchair to another part of the hospital to an x-ray room. The technicians in the x-ray room placed me in a machine similar to a PET scan and completed my x-rays. I was taken back to the Women's center and told that I was done and results would be sent to Dr. Lindsey's office in preparation for my surgery the following morning. I was done for the day and could now prepare myself physically and mentally for surgery.

CHAPTER 29

DAY OF SURGERY (BILATERAL MASTECTOMY)

Tuesday, December 16, 2008-This is the day of my surgery. I was not to have anything via mouth after midnight. I was not to bring anything to the hospital, so I came empty handed with a prayer in my heart. My surgery was scheduled for 7:30 a.m., but I had to report to the main entrance of Northwest Hospital at 5:30 a.m. It was a very early start to the day, but I was ready! I checked in at the front desk then was instructed to go to the level of the hospital where surgery is conducted. The nurse had me undress and put my hospital gown on. She then proceeded with all the standard preparations for surgery.

For a moment, I reminded myself that I was going to come back from this surgery without my breasts. I knew it was for my own good, but it is always difficult facing this kind of challenge. I realized at that moment that sometimes one has to experience great pain in order to gain immense joy. I knew that eliminating this cancer, would give me my life back. I really wanted to live again. I reconciled this loss in my mind one final moment then prepared myself mentally for this experience.

Dr. Harland came in on schedule to greet me, assured me that everything was going to be just fine…and then told me she'd see me in surgery. Dr. Lindsey's assistant came in to place markings on my breasts then she was gone. The Anesthesiologists came in to introduce themselves and said they would make sure they put me to sleep, but better than that, assured me that I'd wake up as well! (smile) They brought a bit of humor to my anxieties!(smile) My dear friend from my church, Evangelist Barbara Colson met us at the hospital about 6:00 a.m. I thought that was extraordinarily thoughtful of her to meet us so early in the morning. She's a real friend and dear sister in the Lord. Paul left out of the room to give her time to visit with me before surgery. It was so good to see her. She shared encouraging words with me, prayed with me, and left my room. Paul came back in and sat patiently until the team of technicians came in to get me and take me away to the operating room. He looked noticeably nervous. I told him I would be fine. He gave me a kiss and left.

I remember hearing the doctors talking to me in the operating room and getting me situated on the operating table...I remember nothing else.

Paul told me later that Dr. Lindsey, Tammie, her PA, and Dr. Harland all came to the waiting area outside the surgical area to let him know how well my surgery went and to let him know that I did well. That was most encouraging news for him. I don't know how long I was in the recovery room...but I think I got to my private room at approximately 3:00 p.m. I remember hearing Paul's voice, and it was the best voice I'd heard since the early morning. Evangelist Colson was still there in my room and it was so good to see and hear her as well. Oh my goodness, she stayed with me from 6:00 a.m. until mid afternoon. What a dedicated friend! I loved her for being there with me and Paul. She gave me a hug and kiss and left. I thanked her for her love and support in my hour of need.

As Evangelist Colson left my room, I remember for the first time...quickly reaching down to feel my chest to see if I had breasts...and unfortunately, they were both gone. There was a moment of sadness that came over me. It was like I'd not only lost a part of my body, but a part of my spirit. Even though I knew I would lose my breasts, I still experienced a moment of emptiness! My emotions overwhelmed me and reality set in. I shed some tears quietly. Paul thought I was in severe pain. I was literally speechless. I prayed softly to the Lord and thanked him for bringing me out of the surgery successfully. I prayed that all my cancer was removed. Then I asked the Lord to help me deal with this extraordinary loss. I felt a calm and peace like I'd not felt since learning of my cancer. I remember being so glad the surgery was all over. Now the real healing process could take place!

Dana and Brittanie came to the hospital to spend time with me, and sleep with me if necessary. Paul was there with me non-stop. He would go home to take care of our dogs, then faithfully come right back to be by my side. How comforting it was to have my family with me. My stay at the hospital would be 3-4 days. The afternoon consisted of round the clock care from my doctors and nurses...the finest medical care ever! I went through a routine of exercises that included; getting me up periodically to use the restroom, providing adequate use of my muscles, legs and arms, and blowing into a respiratory gadget that measured my breathing capability. I had a pump surgically taped to the front of my chest that allowed me to systematically release morphine medication into my system as needed for pain. That was a most needed source of pain relief at this point in my recovery.

I would press the button often to release pain medication. I had other tubes that ran underneath the area where my breasts were and they were attached along each side of my waist. Attached to these tubes were two plastic drainage bulbs on both sides below my waist. This drainage process was called the Jackson Pratt Drainage System. Into these bulbs drained body fluids (consisting of blood cells) from my body as a result of surgery. The nurses would come in periodically to *milk* and empty these bulbs, then record the measurement of fluid via cubic centimeters (cc's).

Dr. Harland and Tammie visited me once, sometimes twice a day to make sure all was going well. Dr. Harland assured me that they were able to remove all of the cancer. I would not know the details of the surgery and Pathology reports until I returned to her office days later for my follow up visit. Dr. Harland asked if I wanted to go home tomorrow (Thursday), and I gladly said…YES! She smiled and eagerly signed my release papers to let me go home the following morning.

Evangelist Vinson called me the day before I left to go home. It was so good to hear her voice! She wanted to come out to visit me, but was combating allergies and a cold. I advised her to stay home and recover. I told her I was comforted just to receive a call from her! How thrilling it was to talk with her. She was one of the last voices I heard on the Sunday before my surgery, as she shared with me what to expect. She and I talked for awhile. I assured her that all went well with my surgery and I looked forward to the healing process. She asked me to expect a floral arrangement to be delivered to my hospital room. Right on schedule, a couple of hours after I spoke with her, the most radiant and beautiful floral planter was delivered. It really made my day. I couldn't have been happier!

The day before I left the hospital, I received a visit from two very sweet ladies who represented Northwest's Breast Cancer support group called *Ladies of the Promise.* They came by to bring me a bag of nice goodies and gifts. One thing that touched me more than any one item in their gift bag was a stuffed animal, which was a panda bear. On the arm of the bear was a pink breast cancer bracelet symbolizing the fight for the cure of breast cancer. I held the animal close to my chest and became quite emotional. I later read the flyer inside the gift bag and learned this was not any stuffed animal.

The animal was designed to conform to your body after breast surgery. The bear therapeutically is held underneath the arm and side as a soft healing source for the patient. How amazing and comforting! The ladies informed me that their business cards were included in my gift pack, and I could call them anytime if I needed someone to talk to or simply needed support of any kind. I was so impressed and sincerely touched by their thoughtfulness and gesture of love.

CHAPTER 30
GOING HOME FROM THE HOSPITAL AND THE AFTERMATH

Thursday, December 18, 2008-I cannot tell you how happy I was to go home! I got up early that morning to freshen up and get myself ready. Paul and Brittanie came to pick me up. I was just as glad to see them as they were to see me. The nurse came in to review all my aftercare papers and instructions. She also instructed me on how to care for my drains and tubes. After she answered my questions concerning my aftercare, she went to order a wheelchair to take me downstairs to the car. I was so glad to have her as my releasing nurse. She was a pleasure to be with during my stay.

I could not be more appreciative of this Northwest Hospital family, the finest team of healthcare professionals in the world. It was somewhat reminiscent of 29 years ago when I'd given birth to Dana at Northwest. Like then, I was treated with such special care!

Friday, December 19, 2008-This is my first day home after surgery. I experienced tremendous pain, but was grateful that I had filled my prescriptions prior to my surgery. I had the tedious task of *milking* my tubes and draining my bodily fluid into drainage bulbs attached to my waist. This was a procedure that the nurses performed in the hospital. I wanted to detach the morphine pump that was attached to my chest. It was so uncomfortable. I routinely milked my tubes and measured my drainage bulbs, documenting my cc counts of fluid at least 3 times a day.
My bulbs were still showing blood in the fluid. I had to continue this process until my fluids showed a clear apple color.

I was so glad to be at home in my own bed. Paul gathered a number of pillows to put behind me and around me to help cushion my chest and underarm area. I could only sleep on my back. How uncomfortable it was. Similar to my chemotherapy treatment, there was nothing I could do about the lack of sleep and discomfort, so I dealt with it the best I could. There was no longer a need to complain. The worst of my worries were behind me. I could only thank God that he saw me through this phase of my journey successfully!

Tuesday, December 23, 2008-I have my follow up appointment with Dr. Lindsey. This is a somewhat difficult appointment, one week after surgery. I am very sore and in some pain. I am managing my pain quite well with medications. However, it is somewhat awkward getting dressed and going to the doctor with these tubes and drainage bulbs attached to my sides. Dr. Lindsey examined my chest area and complimented me on how well my surgical area looked. Of course the precise incisions and success of the procedure, clearly was complimentary of her work. I was concerned about how confining the stitches made me feel. I had many questions for her. I was also concerned about the tenderness I felt of the skin on my chest, and the burning sensation. She said that reaction is as a result of the healing process.

I will experience this feeling for sometime throughout the next few weeks of healing.

I was instructed to use no creams, oils, or moisturizers to the chest until it was healed. She explained that the skin is an organ, and it needs to breathe in order for it to heal. Looking ahead, I had questions concerning my upcoming radiation treatment. Dr. Lindsey advised me to consult with Dr. Harland when I had my follow up appointment with her. Each of my doctors played an intricate role in my aftercare process. It was sometimes difficult to determine which of my symptoms related to which of my doctors. Dr. Lindsey asked me to continue to rest and not exert myself unnecessarily. We wished each other a Merry Christmas and I proceeded to schedule my appointment for the following week. I would need to see the doctor or her PA at least once a week to update my progress and determine when my tubes and drains would be removed from my body. I could not wait!

CHAPTER 31

CHRISTMAS DAY AND NEW YEAR'S EVE

Thursday, December 25, 2008-Christmas day! I was quite emotional at Christmas this year. This is my favorite holiday of the year. I was able to decorate my home so beautifully weeks prior to my surgery. Paul always handled the decorations on the outside of the house. I would spend hours sitting in my living room taking in the sights of all the lovely decorations and whisper prayers thanking God for sparing my life to see this Christmas. I thanked him that my cancer did not consume my body and cause my fatal end. How I praise and glorify the Lord for this opportunity to enjoy this Christmas with my family!

This year, it was the responsibility of my girls and Paul to prepare Christmas dinner and invite only a few guests. I was only up to entertaining my family this year and not others. I had very limited mobility and was still experiencing some pain. As a result, I was unable to be a gracious hostess. It was just good to be with family. We ordered honey baked ham and a turkey breast. My daughters prepared all the side dishes to accompany it. Brittanie prepared a fantastic 3 layer strawberry cake for desert, and Dana prepared her specialty…cheesecake. It was all so delicious. I was proud of them stepping into the role that I always performed. It was nice to sit back and receive royal treatment. (smile)

My granddaughter, Jordynn had been away in Durham, N.C. with her father, Carl while I was recuperating from surgery.
She and Carl came home Christmas Eve, to spend Christmas with Brittanie and our family. It was so good to see her. I'd missed her so much! I could not wait for her to return home with us once I was feeling better.

Christmas morning got off to a great start, with the opening of many gifts for Jordynn, along with her dad, Brittanie, Paul and myself. Jordynn was pleasantly surprised to have her Godmothers come by the house and bring more gifts for her to open. Jordynn tumbled through the many gifts, not quite sure what all of it meant but loving the attention! Later that morning, Dana and Amaya came over...and the gift opening continued for Amaya with a shiny new bicycle. We enjoyed seeing the grands' faces light up with so much fun!

Janise, my stepdaughter, her husband Brian, our son-in-law, along with Zebria, and Zoe, our granddaughterss, left to go out of town to be with their parents in North Carolina for the holiday. If they had been in town, it would have been an even larger family fest of toys, games, and fun. We would extend our celebration with them when they returned home.

My sister, Lorraine and her two children, Kenya and Dwayne came over to join us for dinner. Derron, Dana's boyfriend came later to join us. So we were all gathered together, along with our grands and Carl. We had a touching family prayer around the table and everyone enjoyed themselves, eating, laughing, watching movies and having so much fun! Christmas 2008 was a special day for me. I thanked God for sending His Son, and giving me another chance at LIFE!

Wednesday, December 31, 2008-Like so many others, it has always been my family's tradition to attend New Year's Eve services at my church to welcome in the New Year. It is a wonderful night of preaching, singing, testimonials, and celebration! However, due to my illness and inability to go out, Paul, Dana, Brittanie, Amaya, Jordynn, Zebria, Zoe and myself all saw the New Year in with prayer surrounding my bed. It was very emotional. They didn't go out to church. They all just stayed home to be with me. It was a very special prayer time and everyone cried. How wonderful to see 2009 come in so peacefully with my family gathered together. The year 2008 was a most challenging year for me with my fight with breast cancer. But I vowed to make 2009 a most rewarding year.

It would be a year of anticipation for me to give back to the community of breast cancer survivors. I also wanted to help further the research that would someday find a cure to this dreadful disease. I am so excited about this mission and all the Lord has in store for me!

CHAPTER 32

POST BREAST RESTORATION PROCEDURES

Tuesday, January 6, 2009-This was my follow up visit with Dr. Lindsey. Tammie, Dr. Lindsey's PA was there to assist me, along with Marsha, who is an assistant in the office. Marsha and I sat and talked extensively while waiting for Tammie to come into the room. Tammie had to assist another patient who needed her attention. Marsha and I bonded in friendship with each of my visits. I really looked forward to seeing her each week.

I have to share a funny experience that I had with Marsha at the doctor's office.

I'd mentioned before, how I was experiencing an irritating itching sensation on my chest. It was becoming more and more unbearable. Unable to take this discomfort any longer, I got a bottle of olive oil I had at home. Everyone knows that olive oil is a healthy substance that is used internally to heal various conditions. People cook with it as a spray and a supplement for various foods. The religious community uses it widely throughout churches to anoint the head of individuals, and pray for their various needs. The oil is a substance that some Christians use as a point of contact to pray to God and receive power. With all these valued uses of oil, I felt it wouldn't hurt if I rub some on my chest to soothe this irritated sensation. Well, I couldn't have been more wrong in this case! (smile) I'd only applied this oil once, earlier in the week.

I thought with the showers I'd taken, there would be no traces of it. WRONG! While Marsha was examining me, she saw this oily residue on my chest and was startled as to what it was. When I told her what I'd done, she nearly died! She said I was not to put any kind of creams or oils on my chest. She was unable to examine me properly due to oil build up all over my skin. I was so sorry, and felt really silly for doing something like this. Marsha and I laughed hilariously! I could not have been more embarrassed at my naivety. You can bet, I will never apply oil to my skin again until I'm healed. To see the expression on Marsha's face was priceless! (smile)

Tammie came into the room and saw that my drains were still not draining clear fluid as they should. She realized that I had not been *milking* my tubes properly.

I was again instructed on the proper way to drain the tubes and it made all the difference in my progress. How I wished I'd done it correct previously. I didn't want anything else to hinder my healing process. I was so looking forward to having those bothersome tubes and drainage bulbs taken out. I had to go another week before that would happen. Oh well, I figured I'd come this far, what's another week?! I was happy that I was healing nicely and on schedule. That was great news!

Tuesday, January 13, 2009-Finally, this is my appointment with Dr. Lindsey's PA, Tammie to have my tubes and drainage bulbs removed. The drainage bulbs were now draining clear fluid and looked very good. Tammie examined my drains and saw that they were at the adequate level of cubic centimeters (cc's) at 10-15 cc's on each bulb.

Tammie had Marsha to remove the tubes and bulbs. I didn't know what to expect. My chest was still somewhat sore, so I was hoping and praying that it would not be a procedure that would hurt my sutures. Marsha started the process of removing my tubes. After snipping away a few sutures surrounding the tubes, she asked me to take deep breaths. Between one of those breaths, I'm not sure when she did it, but she pulled them out of each side underneath my arms. It was a strange sensation. I could feel a quick rippling feeling in my chest. It is very hard to explain, but I was relieved. It did not hurt at all! What a relief!

CHAPTER 33

PAUL AND I CELEBRATE OUR WEDDING ANNIVERSARY- FOLLOW UP WITH DR. LINDSEY AND DR. HARLAND

Wednesday, January 21, 2009-This is my 31st wedding anniversary! How exciting, but I spent it at Dr. Lindsey's office beginning the first of my breast tissue expanders inflation process. This would be the first day of a weekly procedure to have needles filled with saline solution injected into each of my breast ports to inflate my breasts. This process was in preparation for my reconstruction surgery.

I had no idea that during my bilateral surgery, I had ports inserted into my breast areas similar to the port that was surgically placed in my chest for chemotherapy access. The ports were used for the injection of saline into my breasts. Thank goodness I had a numbing cream called lidocaine to apply to the area around my ports that would eliminate pain from the stick of the needle. Numbing this area made my weekly visits more comfortable. Each injection would require 60 cc's of saline solution into each breast. As weeks progressed, my breasts would increase in size and would become somewhat sore after each injection. I was instructed to use the same pain reliever and muscle spasm relaxer that I used immediately following my mastectomy surgery. Those pills really did the trick. I endured these weekly procedures with very little or no excessive pain.

Thank goodness for the Lord taking care of me during this phase of my treatments.

On this same day was my final follow up appointment with Dr. Harland following my bilateral mastectomy. She was as bubbly as always and we hugged and kissed reminiscing about my first visit to her June 9, when I learned of my diagnosis of my breast cancer. She applauded my progress, commended my positive spirit, and asked that I make an appointment to come back and see her in 6 months for a follow-up checkup. I could not stop the tears from flowing and shared with her that I could not have made it through this journey without her love, encouragement, and assurance that I would make it through all of this and be alright. I couldn't see then (June 9, 2008), what the Lord had in store for me on this day. I was actually feeling wonderful...but as quickly as we hugged and said our goodbyes...I could feel the pain slowly returning from my breast tissue expander injections just an hour or two earlier. How nice it was to visit with her again. Her spirit was infectious! I then had to quickly leave her office, get home, and take pain medications.

But remember...this is my wedding anniversary day! Paul, being the romantic that he is, would not let this day go with only a succession of doctors' visits and not celebrate our special day. He surprised me when I got home from the doctors' office with a take-out dinner from Bighorn Steakhouse of a full dinner,

minus the candle lights! I was feeling too uneasy from the procedure earlier that day from the doctor and it was quite difficult to relax with an anniversary dinner. He was so sweet to wait until after I slept off my medication, then we were able to enjoy dinner together that evening! It was as sweet and romantic as any girl could wish for. He even ordered my favorite fruit basket from one of my favorite decorative fruit shops…"Fruitful Art Arrangements."
It was spectacular! I couldn't have been happier on this special day! For those few hours, I completely forgot all about my condition and what I'd gone through. I did, however celebrate the day I'd met Paul, and we joined in marriage…31 years ago. He is the best!

CHAPTER 34
HERCEPTIN TREATMENTS RESUMED-ECKO CARDIO TESTS

Friday, January 23, 2009-I visited GEORGIA CANCER CENTER to resume my Herceptin treatments. It was so good to see everyone on staff again. I had not seen them since November 2008 when I received my last treatment prior to surgery. I visited with Dr. Sharian. He was very pleased with my Pathology report. He said my report was one of the best reports he'd seen of any of his cancer patients. He asserted that there might be a possibility that I would not have to undergo radiation treatment! I really needed to hear this great news! Paul and I nearly shouted for joy!

We were so overwhelmed by that news, because it had been my prayer not to have to undergo radiation. However, he said we would wait until the end of February and set up a consultation appointment with the Radiologist. Once the Radiologist received my records and give me a thorough examination, he would be able to make a better judgment. The Radiologist would make the final decision if radiation treatment was needed. All I could do was continue to pray that I would bypass this portion of the treatment process. Dr. Sharian set up a routine follow up appointment with Dr. Reid, my Cardiologist for an echo cardio exam and chest x-rays at Fairway Fayette Hospital.

Tuesday, January 27, 2009-This was the day of my appointment with the Cardiologist and x-rays at Fairway Fayette Hospital.

The Cardiologist confirmed that there was fluid retention under my skin in my chest. This was normal following this type of surgery. The fluid retention contributed to some of the painful discomfort and tenderness I was experiencing on my chest. The healing process would eliminate this tenderness as time progressed. After a follow-up visit with Dr. Lindsey's office, I was relieved to know that I could now use a soothing crème to help relieve the tenderness on my chest. I continued my weekly visits to Dr. Lindsey's office for my breast tissue expander procedures.

Friday, January 30, 2009-I visited the GEORGIA CANCER CENTER and was able to again resume my Herceptin treatment and continued with them every 3 weeks. I would continue with these treatments through September 2009.

After September, I would only need to go to the GEORGIA CANCER CENTER every quarter for the next 3 years. While I will be so happy to be done with the treatments, I will desperately miss the staff. They had been a life-line for me throughout this journey. I couldn't have done it without them! They have all been the kindest medical staff team I've known throughout my illness.

Wednesday, February 11, 2009-This was a pretty exciting day for me. I was able to start back driving. It felt so great and gave me my independence back. I didn't have to depend on Paul and Brittanie to chauffeur me to and from the doctor's offices. It was quite liberating!

CHAPTER 35

CONSULTATION WITH ONCOLOGY RADIOLOGIST TO BEGIN RADIATION THERAPY TREATMENTS

Tuesday, March 3, 2009-This was my first appointment/consultation with my Radiologist, Dr. Carla Chu at the South Fulton Radiation Oncology Services office. She was such a confident young doctor who came into the office to see me. After reviewing all my many CT, PET scans, MRI exams, Oncology reports, Pathology reports, and all x-rays, she concluded that I would still need to undergo radiation treatment. She stated furthermore that she would need to radiate my left chest area and the left side of my neck for approximately 5 ½ weeks. My heart dropped 10 feet!

I was so sure I would not have to undergo this portion of the treatment process. I had an intense confrontation with Dr. Chu and requested that she consult with Dr. Sharian again to make sure. My mind was so made up on not having to undergo this treatment. She could see my intensity and determination. She assured me that she would consult with her other Radiologist colleagues. She informed me that the Radiologists all meet every Wednesday to consult on various patient's cases and she would discuss my case with them. Their next meeting would be Wednesday, March 11th. Trina, Dr. Chu's nurse gave me an armful of material to read to familiarize myself with the radiation process. It explained what to expect during and after the procedure. I walked out of the office vowing not to read it. I really didn't think it would apply to me. I didn't want to have to go through this at all.

I walked to my car very disappointed that radiation was recommended for me. I suddenly became so depressed. I felt the warm tears on my face begin to flow again.

I was set to go on a vacation getaway alone on Thursday, March 12th. I was so looking forward to finally getting away and resting my mind. I'd wanted to get away since I learned of my diagnosis June of 2008. Radiation or no radiation, I knew I had to getaway! My mind was about to go into a mental melt down and I needed this time. I asked the Lord, to please relax my mind and let me try to process all the medical and emotional experiences I'd undergone.

Wednesday, March 11, 2009-Dr. Chu called me back and confirmed that her colleagues agreed that radiation treatment would be recommended in my case. I finally accepted but told her I would be going away for a few days and would call her when I returned to town. She understood and asked me to have a great vacation and get a lot of rest. Trust me that was my plan!

Thursday March 12th-Sunday March 15, 2009-I had the most beautiful and relaxing vacation at Midway

Gardens. It is only 45 minutes south of Atlanta, and it was the perfect time of year without all the tourists and crowds. I loved my drive there. It relaxed my mind. I saturated my spirit with praise and worship music along with a variety of very relaxing music. It was a getaway just for me! Paul would have gone with me, but he wanted me to have this time alone. He would go the following week to visit with his stepmother in South Carolina. We both needed time away for ourselves. We had experienced 6-8 months of pure mental and emotional exhaustion. We owed this time to ourselves. Midway Gardens is such a beautiful resort. The atmosphere and late winter scenery was just what I needed. I enjoyed a wonderful communion with the Lord…and I know he enjoyed me!

CHAPTER 36
ONCOLOGIST CONFIRMS NEED FOR RADIATION TREATMENT- DISAPPOINTING NEWS

Friday, March 20, 2009-This was my routine Herceptin treatment at the GEORGIA CANCER CENTER. Dr. Sharian visited with me during this time before my treatment and told me that he agreed with my recommendation of radiation treatment therapy. I was so disappointed that he agreed with it. I had always looked to Dr. Sharian as my saving grace. I looked to him as a type of *savior*. He, with the leading of the Lord, rescued my life from a terminal illness that could have been the end for me. His treatments, recommendations and care for my life were extraordinary!

When he confirmed the need for radiation, my heart again just dropped. Nevertheless, I valued his opinion in all medical decisions for my life and I would not deter from his counsel. It was imperative for him to share with me his convictions and basis for agreeing to radiation treatment.

What he said to me troubled my mind terribly! He explained that I had 4 risk factors in determining my need for radiation. He said I was... 1.) HER 2 Neu positive which is one of the most serious and aggressive forms of breast cancer in women. This status contributed to my treatment of Herceptin. He explained that HER 2 Neu positive patients will have a faster chance of recurrence of cancer without radiation treatment...and Lord knows I didn't want that to happen. 2.) I am premenopausal. I had not had a menstrual cycle since being diagnosed with cancer, June 9, 2008. I don't know if it was the shock of learning of my cancer that my mental blockers just shut down and could not process my cycle or what. I completely forgot that I had not had a menstrual cycle...it just didn't happen, and it didn't even dawn on me that I hadn't had one until halfway through my chemo treatments when I was asked by Dr. Harland during my visit with her the end of August 2008. It was amazing...no more menstrual trauma! YAY! 3.) I was considered, by Dr. Chu's terminology, *Neo-adjuvant*. This means that I had my chemotherapy treatment before surgery. The chemo shrunk and destroyed all tumors that existed before surgery. Dr. Chu insisted that they did not know or have any way of knowing what tumors and/or lymphnodes existed before surgery and she could not determine which of those tumors/lymphnodes that were positive with cancer cells and the degree of cancer that existed in those cells. 4.) Finally, I am Estrogen Negative, which means I have not yet had Estrogen or hormone treatment.

Dr. Sharian intimately shared with me that he could not, consciously, not recommend radiation treatment and take a chance on my cancer returning. He said he could not disagree with the Radiologists recommendation. We seemed to have intensely discussed this decision with great passion. I explained to him that if I had the radiation treatment administered, it would delay my reconstruction surgery to restore my breasts for another 6-9 months...possibly a year. Having my breasts surgically restored meant so much to me...the sooner the better. He finally shared with me that at my age, 56, I have statistically only 25 more years of life (since the average woman only lived until age 75).

He said I could live a good quality life for another 25 years with the treatment of radiation as opposed to not receiving it at all.

I disappointedly received Dr. Sharian's words and walked away from his office to the treatment room for my Herceptin treatment. It was such a depressing day for me in the treatment room, which is normally a fun-filled time with the nurses. They make anyone's terrible day turn into a delight. I could only sit and cry quietly to myself and try to not let anyone see. I am normally one of their perkiest patients, but not today! Karen, one of the nurses in the treatment room, noticed that I was looking unusually depressed. She was one that would make all of the patients' day seem brighter, even when they were not feeling well. She always had the words, jovial attitude, and personality to enlighten anyone's day!

I remember Karen's words to me that really pierced my heart. She said "now you just need to get a grip and cheer yourself on up!" "You have done so well and have come such a long way, and you need to see this treatment to the end!" She further shared with me that there are patients that come through this room with stage 4 cancer who live on to lead wonderful lives, and others with stage 1 and 2 cancer who don't make it. She made me feel like the most blessed person in the world. She encouraged me to continue with my treatment, even if radiation was my next step. I will never forget Karen's encouraging words. She'll never know what it meant to me!

I knew I would be alright. After all, I'd just returned from a fantastic vacation and was emotionally prepared for any decisions the doctors would make. I finally had to reconcile in my mind that I had come this far in my journey and once I completed the radiation treatment, I would be closer to ending this whole process. I knew the Lord was still with me every step of the way, I would continue to pray for peace…and always remember Karen's words that day that helped make the difference!

CHAPTER 37

BREAST RESTORATION PROCEDURES RESUMED

Wednesday, March 25, 2009-Since radiation therapy treatment had been decided in my case, Dr. Lindsey had a critical decision to make. She was possibly two thirds through the completion of my breast tissue expander inflation phase. It was important for me to complete the injections of the saline solution into the breast expanders because without their completion, the damage of radiation would deplete the consistency and quality of their staying in place in my chest in preparation for my final reconstruction surgery. Dr. Chu and Dr. Lindsey thoroughly discussed my case.

With the sensitivity of time lost before starting my radiation, Dr. Chu decided that it would do no harm to have Dr. Lindsey continue with the inflation process of my breast expanders. However, Dr. Lindsey's office would need to contact the Radiologists immediately when the breast expander process was done so that preparations and tests for radiation could be set up and administered following the process.

This phase of the process had become somewhat aggravating for me. I knew the urgency of starting my radiation treatment with time being of the essence. I wanted to go ahead with treatment as soon as possible. I would go weekly for these breast tissue expander injections. I needed a total of 900 cc's of saline solution in each of my breasts. Dr. Lindsey's team was very accommodating and commended my patience in the process. Little did they know I was becoming more and more impatient with each visit. I really wanted to get the radiation phase of this journey over so I could finalize my reconstruction surgery.

Upon my last visit to Dr. Lindsey's office for my final breast tissue expander inflation procedure, I then learned that I would need to have my implants surgically inserted before radiation therapy could start. I knew I needed implants in place, but I thought this was done with the final reconstruction surgery. I did not understand the medical process of what procedure took precedence over the other in moving to the next step in this whole reconstruction process. I was thrilled to learn that once the implants were in place and the breast expanders were removed, that would be my final step before radiation treatment. The implants would be held intact in the breast cavity wall, with the hopes that radiation would cause little or no shrinkage or damage.

Ok, now the only thing left to do with Dr. Lindsey's office, at this point, was to set up a date for my surgery to insert my implants and remove my breast tissue expanders. Marsha, my dear friend and assistant to Dr. Lindsey, took me into a room and scheduled my appointment for surgery for April 27th. I was scheduled to have pre-op done on April 22nd. It felt so good to finally have my next phase moving and steering me towards radiation. Please let's just get it over with so I can get this radiation done and move on with my life! I can finally say that my zeal for "patience" was finally back!

CHAPTER 38
MOTHER BERNICE MURPHY- WHAT A VISIT!

Friday, April 3, 2009-This was a wonderful day of fellowship and love when I visited with a dear Mother of our church, Mother Bernice Murphy. Mother Murphy epitomized the spirit of faith in its most vibrant state. She was diagnosed with breast cancer approximately 5 or 6 years ago. Her faith dictated her life and prayer was her guide. She did not allow the seriousness of her diagnosis to determine her quality of life. When the doctors told her of her cancer and her prognosis, she decided then that she would wait on God to heal her body and not agree to any traditional form of cancer treatments whatsoever. Our church members watched Mother Murphy attend services week after week with that golden smile as only she could give. Whether in pain or agony, she always smiled and exhorted a word of healing to whomever was near. She knew God would heal her and she didn't want to suffer with destructive chemicals of chemotheraphy or radiation.

I would speak with Mother Murphy at Bible studies and at church on Sundays and she would always declare the *Glory of God* and testify that she was going on with the Lord and nothing would turn her faith from trusting Him to heal her. I shared my love with Mother Murphy and basked in her presence...so full of faith...not realizing then that one day we would share not only our love but our illnesses as well. When she learned of my illness, she would only smile at me and tell me... "God is able!" I knew then that she wanted me to trust God for my healing. While I knew God as a healer, I chose to accept traditional medical care and treatment. She understood my choice and prayed with me accordingly. She later told me that the Lord had shown her...from the day I was diagnosed, that I would be just fine. I was at peace with her words and went on with my treatments and surgeries.

As time passed by, and the years progressed, I saw Mother become weaker, yet her smile gleamed wide as ever. She moved a little slower, since she was fighting various other illnesses in her body as a result of her cancer. I would go up to her and hug her...and her words to me would always be... "Sister Baldwin, God is able." She spoke prophetic words when given the opportunity at church, and shared with different ones personally the power of God. What a praying woman of God she was! As Mother's condition worsened and the cancer took its toll on her physical body, she would attend services, but she sat in the balcony of the church where most of us who were recovering from surgery or illnesses sat. This allowed us not to surround ourselves with crowds of people. Sometimes the many hugs would be too crushing on our already frail bodies. I too sat in the balcony while I was undergoing chemotherapy and could not communicate with the members for fear of compromising my immune system. I would see Mother Murphy from a distance from my side of the balcony to the other side where she sat. We would wave at each other and she'd blow me a kiss! What affection I felt for her as we both suffered in our own silence. She taught me so much about faith and patience.

As she became immobile and was unable to walk, she continued to attend services and I was unable to see her as often. She never wavered in her spirit as she faithfully pressed her way through much pain to be a part of the fellowship. So it was on this day, April 3rd, that I was finally able to go visit with her at her home.

I'd just had a visit with Dr. Lindsey's office, undergoing one of my breast tissue expander procedures. I was in slight pain, but was determined to see Mother Murphy.

Our visit was as though the clouds were rolled back in my life and her presence allowed me to view my life more clearly. How refreshing it was to sit next to her while she struggled to the bed after her shower.
I could see how the fluid build-up in her chest, arm, and facial areas were quite visible. She wore a glow on her face that I'd not seen before. Her smile and candor was quick and sharper than ever. We spent

hours talking about the Lord. We talked about what the Lord had done for us in each of our lives and made plans for our futures. One of our plans was a long lost promise we'd made to one another that she would teach Paul and I how to can and jar fruits and vegetables. This was a desire of ours that we'd talked about doing in the past. Mother Murphy grinned with this childish grin and said how excited she was to come out to my home and how we would sit around and can and jar fruit all afternoon! She never once acted like a woman whom the doctors had just weeks before, announced that she had only days or weeks to live. How my heart was in awe at her stamina, her grace, her faith!

She wanted me to read any scriptures out of the Bible that my heart desired. I did. Her favorite scriptures were the ones that spoke on healing…mine were of peace. She laid back in bed and rested with a smile, pondering over the mere power of God's Word. I too smiled that I was there to share it with her, and to know that we both, suffering with breast cancer, were blessed by God's healing power.

She suddenly bounced up off the bed, quickly went into her restroom, and came back out with a box full of goodies that she said that she wanted to give me. She was so happy to have found a wholesale store out in the Douglasville area that gave away toiletries and various hygienic products. She gave me a handful of really nice stuff. She seemed so thrilled to do it...and I was as thrilled to receive it.

She then slowly moved around her room and grabbed this picture from her wallet. It was a picture of a little girl that appeared to be approximately 6 years old. She asked me teasingly if I knew who that little girl was. I didn't have a clue and asked her to tell me. She said it was her at the tender young age of, I believe she said, 7 or 8 years old. How cute she was, and I found it even more adorable that she wanted to share it with me!

Mother Murphy then began to share with me about the health of her nephew, who lived in Tennessee. He was gravely ill, in a coma, and she longed to go and be with him to pray and care for him. We both prayed and agreed that on some level the Lord would touch and save him, and ultimately heal his body.

She shared about her late husband, who gave his life to Lord at the end of his life and this pleased her more than anything in their marriage. She was most proud of the hundreds of souls that she'd brought to the Lord and prayed for their salvation. She shared with me visions the Lord had given her of others' lives that she'd also shared with them. Each experience she shared was extraordinarily powerful. I was so moved by Mother Murphy. Her exhortations made me forget about my own imminent pain from the procedure I'd undergone earlier that day.

It was time for me to leave her. How I wished I could have stayed longer and hear more of her life's experiences. I prayed for her, then she prayed for us both. How magnificent to be with a woman with a heart for the Lord as she had.
It was only 3 weeks after my visit, that we'd received the word that Mother Murphy quietly passed away at her home. I'm told that she left this earth, still reaching out to others sharing the love of God. What a soul, what a life, what a spirit! My faith has been lifted, just by having known her.

CHAPTER 39

BREAST IMPLANT SURGERY

Monday, April 27, 2009-My second of three surgeries is set for today at 1:00 p.m. at Northwest Hospital. It was scheduled to be an outpatient surgery, however due to the fact that I was having such a hard time waking up and staying alert, they kept me overnight. My pain level was minimal compared to my bilateral surgery in December 2008. My implants were in, I was able to go home the next day and all was well with my health! I was so happy to finally prepare for radiation. As strange as that sounds and knowing all the negative effects from radiation to come, I was prepared for its impact and aftermath.

It could not be nearly as bad as what I suffered with chemotherapy. My focus now was to heal in my body from surgery and move forward.

I continued with my Herceptin treatment at the GEORGIA CANCER CENTER every 3 weeks on schedule. I went to Dr. Lindsey's office for my follow up visit one week after my surgery and it was amazing what a fantastic job she did on my chest. The job she did removing my breast tissue expanders and inserting my implants was awesome. They looked marvelous! All systems were a *go* for radiation. I called Dr. Chu's office and they immediately set my appointment for CT scans, x-rays, and planning in preparation for radiation treatment.

CHAPTER 40
PREPARATION FOR RADIATION TREATMENT

Thursday, May 21, 2009-This is my first appointment with the South Fulton Radiation Oncology Services office for my CT scan, and x-rays. A wonderful nurse technician serviced me and took care of my scan and x-rays. The process in preparation for radiation was fascinating. My body was marked with X's and markings that would serve as tattoo indicators on my skin. These tattoo indicators allow rays to be projected via radiation equipment that destroys residue of cancer cells. Dr. Chu came in after I was marked and consulted with me to tell me where she would radiate me and the effects of the radiation. She again informed me that my left breast area would be the focus along with my left neck area. She further warned me of the possible effects that radiation would have on my heart and lung organs. However, the team of technicians monitor the process carefully to prevent damage to these organs. Methodically, they focus on those areas needed to prohibit the furtherance of cancer cells, with preventative measures taken to protect vital organs. I felt confident in Dr. Chu's procedures along with my prayers that the Lord would protect my body from unnecessary harm.

Friday, May 22, 2009-I was asked to come into the Radiation office and have my permanent tattoos tacked in place on those strategic pinpoints on my body. Tattoos were placed on my chest area, and the sides of my waist. I could finally say that I was among the *tattooed "in-crowd"*! I teased the technicians and told them I was so disappointed that they didn't tattoo a large dragon on my chest or maybe even a butterfly (smile)! They chuckled then escorted me back to the front office. My radiation treatment was scheduled to start the day after Memorial day, May 26th.

Tuesday, May 26, 2009-This is my first day of radiation treatment. I would be slated to undergo 5 ½ -6 weeks of daily treatments. I marked my calendar for everyday of my treatment. I saw that they would end approximately July 6th. Again, it would end as it began, a couple of days after another holiday…the 4th of July. I would lie on the table each day for treatment, anticipating how my body would react to the burning sensations or skin discoloration. Whatever happened, I would be so prepared for it. I bought aloe vera gel, as recommended by Dr. Chu and applied it to my skin every day and night immediately following each treatment. It was full of menthol, which was cool and soothing to my skin. I prayed that it would continue to serve its purpose when and if my skin became irritated and tender. I was happy to finally start my radiation treatments.

Thursday, June 25, 2009-Four weeks into radiation treatment I began experiencing severe burning and pain under my left arm. My skin had become charcoal black. After my treatment today, Dr. Tindle decided to suspend me from further treatment until Tuesday, June 30th. Along with using aloe vera gel, I was given a prescription for a healing cream called silver sulfadiazine. Its use would prove to soothe the burning that I experienced. It also contained an antibiotic ingredient that would protect the skin from infection. I was instructed to use it 3 times a day, however, I was instructed to not use it 4 hours prior to my radiation treatment. In addition, I had to take a pain med to help ease my discomfort.

Tuesday, June 30, 2009-I used the cream daily as instructed. However, when I went back to the office for treatment, I was still in so much pain. I could hardly lift my left arm, and my skin was still tender to the touch. Once Dr. Chu examined me, she asked that I take a longer break from treatment. I was not only suspended from today's treatment, I was instructed not to return until after the 4th of July Holiday on Monday, July 6th. This initially would have been my completion date for treatment, so it appeared that I would be delayed from completing my treatment now until Monday, July 13th. Oh well, I thought, I'm almost done!

We really needed another break just to get-away and rest. Paul, Amaya and I packed the car up and left the very next day and went to Midway Gardens for a nice few days of rest before the holiday crowd would descend on the beautiful beach, and grounds. We went to the beach, circus, butterfly garden, and just enjoyed the many amenities the resort offered. It was a nice rest and a fun filled weekend!

CHAPTER 41

GEORGIA CANCER CENTER ORDERS ANOTHER CT SCAN

Friday, July 3, 2009-I had to go into the GEORGIA CANCER CENTER for a CT scan that was ordered. At this point in the aftermath of my cancer treatments, this was ordered to assure that no more cancer cells existed. I could only pray to God for great results. This scan meant more to me than any of the others. This marked the end of an era with my cancer and I really wanted to put it behind me. Lord please let me receive a good report!

Friday, July 10, 2009-Carmen, my favorite PA at the GEORGIA CANCER CENTER was waiting for me with a big cheery smile to give me test results on my CT scan. She reviewed all of my lab results which were quite good. She then had a concerned look on her face when she informed me that the CT scan revealed a 9.2 cm mass on my uterus. My mind immediately went blank! This discovery, no matter how discreetly Carmen tried to share it with me along with efforts to keep me calm, did not process well with me. I instantly went into stress-mode and replayed thoughts of my initial cancer discovery in my mind. I couldn't imagine anything else going wrong with my health at this point in my life. Lord knows I'd exemplified the utmost of faith. With the same energy that I chose to stress myself unnecessarily, I used my faith to pray to God for strength and patience through yet another obstacle.

I was determined to achieve my goal of living *cancer free*! Carmen forwarded a copy of the CD of my x-rays to Dr. Yancey's office.

I was scheduled for an appointment to see him for further examination and test results.

CHAPTER 42
LAST DAY OF RADIATION TREATMENT AND THE END OF HERCEPTIN TREATMENT

Monday, July 13, 2009-This is my last day of radiation therapy treatment! YAY! You don't know how thrilled and happy I was! I was seen by Dr. Tindle, since Dr. Chu was on duty at the hospital and was unable to be with me for my final visit. How I wanted her to be there so I could hug her neck and thank her for how comfortable she'd made my treatment visits. Dr. Tindle examined me, gave me a clean bill of health, and released me from their services. I was scheduled to come back to see Dr. Chu in 3 weeks, on July 31st.

This would be for my final exit visit to assure that my skin and breast area were healing properly. The nurse then came into the office to go over aftercare instructions and have me sign release forms. I also received a *certificate of completion*! I was as thrilled to receive this certificate as graduating from any University. Making it through the radiation process was a great accomplishment to me.

Later that morning on this same day, while celebrating my victory of completing my radiation treatments, I received a call from Dr. Yancey's office at exactly 12:00 noon. I was not expecting any further delays for my return to work and seeing all my friends and co-workers again! Dr. Yancey confirmed the mass that was found on my uterus via the CT scan. He stated that the mass needed to be further examined via sonogram at his office on that following Friday, July 17, 2009.

Friday, July 17, 2009-I went to Dr. Yancey's office as requested and had my sonogram exam done. THANK GOD, it was not cancerous. How relieved I was just knowing that the Lord was still hearing my prayers! GOD IS **SO** GOOD!

Friday, September 11, 2009-This was the last day of ALL treatments! This marked the end of a year's treatment of Herceptin. I would no longer have to go back to the cancer treatment rooms for chemo, Herceptin, or any treatments that required accessing my port in my chest. I was so looking forward to Dr. Sharian scheduling my outpatient surgery to have my port in my chest removed.

CHAPTER 43
MY FIRST SPEAKING ENGAGEMENT AS BREAST CANCER SURVIVOR

Saturday, September 12, 2009-An exciting occasion began to happen for me on this day. I was invited to be one of the many speakers at my first Health Fair in Cartersville, Georgia. I was asked to speak as a breast cancer survivor and share my story to a host of other women who might benefit. How glad I was to not only share my story, but to welcome the opportunity to begin helping other women who had fears, concerns and doubts concerning breast cancer. I remembered when I was diagnosed and welcomed the stories of so many women who were there to help me.

It was such a lovely day and an eagerly inquisitive crowd was there to learn more about prevention, care, and treatment of breast cancer. I was graciously welcomed and honored to be a part of such an event.

As the Lord began to open doors for me to speak on various occasions, I was asked to speak at my church Women's Luncheon in the preparation for *Breast Cancer Awareness* month, on September 26, 2009. It was such a lovely affair, where women were all dressed in pink. As the Keynote Speaker, I was asked to share my story. The Lord blessed so many of us during that luncheon. We loved, cried, learned and supported one another in our fight against breast cancer. I was especially happy to have my two daughters, Dana and Brittanie there with me. Their love and support was so special.

I knew this was a turning point for me in my life…the Lord knew exactly what I prayed for all those months lying in bed struggling in pain with my cancer. I asked the Lord to not only allow me to live through this terrible disease, but allow me to minister to others of His healing power! I knew if I was to be healed of cancer, the Lord was the only one to do it. I would never forget what He ministered to me while I was sick in bed day after day, and night after night. The Lord spoke so audibly to me that "He would not only heal me of my cancer, but allow me to stand in the gap for so many who did not have the faith to believe." His spirit penetrated my very being so deeply that I would almost forget that I'd ever been sick.

I was singed with coals of fire, yet glowing in God's perfect light. There is not a more amazing experience than to be one in the spirit with the Lord.

I felt that moment of *oneness* when I ministered to others. What an incredible HIGH!

CHAPTER 44

MY PORT IS SURGICALLY REMOVED FROM MY CHEST - A "CLEAN BILL OF HEALTH"!

Monday, October 12, 2009-This was also a very exciting day for me. I was scheduled for outpatient surgery to have my port removed from my chest. This removal of my port was most symbolic to me. This represented the end of cancer and all cancer treatments. I knew once I had the port removed, I would view it as a bridge that I passed over. A bridge, over tumultuous waters, but I survived it and I could only pray that I would not have to go back over that bridge again. I rested at home after surgery with a smile on my face.

No longer having a port in my chest, to me, represented freedom to live again! Praise the Lord!

Tuesday, October 27, 2009-This was my follow up visit with Dr. Harland. I was so glad to see her again! After all, her office is where I was initially informed of my cancer. I cannot tell you the overwhelming emotion I felt while going through the various tests prior to seeing her again. All the traumatic thoughts I experienced when I first visited her office were there. I remember what was to be a routine visit, turned into a nightmare, but not this time. She and all her nursing assistants were as cordial as always. When she gave me the good news of my chest looking exceptionally well, she and all the office celebrated with me! I shared with Dr. Harland that I was experiencing swelling under my arms, and some discomfort in positioning myself for sleeping.
She assured me that what I was feeling was completely normal and was nothing extraordinary. The slight discomfort experienced from bilateral surgery, eases over time. I felt more relaxed hearing

these comforting words from her. She said I don't need to return for another six months. I held Dr. Harland in my arms and cried so hard. I didn't want to let her go! She was my greatest source of strength to get me through this journey. She was the very first one who held my hand and told me I would be alright and I would get through this horrific time in my life! She was exactly right! She had the same infectious smile on her face that she had the first day I met her and she told me my news of having cancer. Her calming spirit makes one feel that they can get through anything. I left her office feeling *more than a conqueror*! I knew the Lord sent her to me.

She was truly my angel advocating on my behalf! So my story ends with as powerful an impact as it began. I learned to triumph in tragedy. The Word of God has proven true in my life… "that all things work together for good to them that love the Lord." He is always working for our good.

CHAPTER 45
SO WHERE DO I GO FROM HERE... AND WHAT HAVE I LEARNED

So Lord, now what do you want from me? I asked myself that question time and time again after I conquered this test. I cannot explain the joy in my heart I felt after my final examination from my Oncologist once I'd completed chemotherapy and radiation treatments. The words, "cancer free" did not sound sweeter than it did when they were whispered to me. All tests show no more cancer cells evident. I was so relieved of the pain, stress, and agony of this fight. Overcoming cancer is truly a fight. When someone loses their fight and transitions to be with the Lord, they have truly fought a fight as vigorously as a soldier in battle.

    I knew that my life would take on a whole new meaning, and would never be the same. When one lives through a traumatic health crisis, your attitude towards life, ministry, and people changes. I knew I had a new mission in life and more importantly, a new vow to the Lord. My heart was inspired to help others suffering with cancer. I wanted to be there for them, tell them they would be alright, and encourage them to pray to a God that still heals!

    How do I get this word out to the masses? The message being, there is life after much suffering? Writing this book was my first step. I feel that other women who have been diagnosed with breast cancer and those who are feeling a moment of uncertain despair would be strengthened by my own experience. Understanding that everyone experiences life's disappointments differently, we can do what we can to help one's trial a little easier.

The Lord desires to send a message to the world through everyone's life, and His message might be uniquely revealed from one spirit to another. I pray that my plight speaks power to others as it did me. The Lord desires to draw us closer to Him through his love and healing power. His healing power allowed me to see him through his eyes.

Each and every person I have met through my illness has completely changed my life. I became so attentive to every word spoken to me by each individual, so as not to miss the voice of the Lord. Whether by thought, words, or deeds…I absorbed all there was to learn from others. I must say that the Lord has Angels all around us in this life and we must be mindful… as Hebrews 13:2 says, "we must be careful not to entertain angels unawares." Whether someone was a health professional, fellow patient, friend, co-worker, or family member, their lives have touched me in ways unimaginable.

The lessons I have learned on this journey are many. One should never take life for granted. Behind every door is a rainbow with many different aspects of our lives. How we accept and process those experiences are entirely up to us. We can make life as beautiful as it is intended or we can take those experiences and allow them to become a yoke upon our hearts and wear us down. One can never go forward looking down, but can go forward with their head up in the air. I choose to move forward with a new life. I choose to allow the Lord's Will to be my guide. I choose to soar! I finally asked myself, where do I go from here? I'm going to live a life filled with abundance and joy.

There's a huge world out there, and I want to touch everyone in my path...whether through thought, word, or deed. As a Christian, ministry is so important. I plan to minister life in the Lord to everyone who needs Him. The act of ministering has never taken on such meaning as it has for me now. True ministry brings about a change. If I can change someone's life for the better, then I have accomplished my mission the Lord has for me. Throughout my journey, the one scripture that spoke life to me was II Corinthians 4:17 "For our light affliction, which is but for a moment, worketh for us a far more exceeding and eternal weight of glory." Our sufferings on this earth is only for a moment compared to the sufferings of Christ. Certainly He endured the cross for us, a sacrifice we could never repay.

    I am humbled and honored to have been chosen by God to endure such a trial, in my cancer fight. He has proven himself to me to be as comforting in tragedy and as fierce in triumph! One never wants their life to be lived in vain, but lived to the fullest. I intend to do just that!

    ....I pray you will forever "*hear*" the sun shine in your life!

ACKNOWLEDGMENTS

From the time that I was diagnosed with breast cancer, the people in my life have been phenomenal. My family, friends, church family and co-workers have been "God sent". I believe they have always been there, but life-changing experiences like this reveals true hearts. I have learned how to genuinely love people more. One's life changes immensely after an experience like this. I would love to pay tribute to those special spirits.

- **To Evangelist Dr. Carolyn Vinson and Apostle Dr. Thomas Vinson, my extraordinary Pastors.** You were there for me every step of the way. You prayed for me and loved me like no other Pastors could. Evangelist Vinson, your own breast cancer experience paved the way for every test, procedure, and treatment I endured. Thank you for sharing the Lord and your life with me.

- **To Deacon Louvenia Willis.** Your learning of your breast cancer scare opened the door for you to hold my hand and prepare me for the most frightening diagnosis of my life. Thanks for those "first prayers". They meant more than you'll ever know.

- **To my Mother (Lucile Mosley), Father (Johnny Mosley Sr.), my Brothers (Johnny/Charlotte, Larry/Yvonne, Jeffrey, and Lyle/Janis) and Sisters (Evelyn/Ervin, Brenda/Tony, Sr., Lorraine, and Barbara).** You all taught me the roots of my spiritual growth. Thank you for your love and support.

- **To my brother Pastor Larry Mosley and his lovely wife, Yvonne.** You were there visiting me regularly, praying with me, and making sure I was alright. Thank you so much.

- **A special thank you to my oldest sister, Evelyn Myers.** Your hours of proofreading notes, revisions, and the time you donated to my book was priceless. Thanks for helping to make this a smooth read.

- **To Evangelist Ethel Womack.** You were like my natural Sister, and the best friend ever. You were there when I needed you most. Thanks for the shoulder.

- **To Valerie High,** one of the most talented playwrights and writers of our times. Your resourceful writing expertise and advice was invaluable. How can I say…thanks?

- **To Elder Denise Jarrett** for taking the time out of your busy schedule to help proofread my book. Your expertise and advice was most needed and sincerely appreciated. Thanks for being a friend and mentor.

- **To Ferrinnia (Toni) High and Kim Bashir.** You two ladies were the first to tell me that I need to keep a journal of my cancer experience and later publish it into a book. Thanks for providing the journals to capture my notes.

- **To Antoinette McKenzie** for your love and support each time I e-mailed you apologizing for my being out sick, unable to fulfill my duties

on the "Announcements" team. Your thoughts and prayers were always appreciated.
- **To my Co-workers of GCAPP.** I couldn't have made it through this illness without your support. I'll never forget my "red survival bag" with gifts galore. I took it with me everyday of my treatments to remind me of you.
- **To all of my Highpoint Christian Tabernacle church family.** You are all so very incredible and giants amongst spiritual giants.
- **To Shelia Barnes** who also survived Cancer. You are one of the most praying, full of encouragement Sisters I know. Thank you for breathing God's Word into me when I needed it most.
- **To Shontell Hughes**. You were there to serve in my place during Baptism and pray for me when I couldn't resume my duties at church. I thank you for your faithfulness and diligence.
- **To Dee Dee Moltz** (from my husband's former job, Sun Chemical) who is also a breast cancer survivor. You called me weekly to check on me when I was sick and forecasted to the day of each chemo treatment, when I would be sick

and even lose my hair. I love you for caring and your support.

- **To those of you who went online to the American Cancer Society's site** and purchased the fanciest hats/caps to cover my bald head...Johnny and Charlotte Mosley, Evelyn Myers, Joanne Trammell, Rose Saxon, Tina Harrington, Toni High, and Gladys White.

- **To Wilhelmina Garrison and "Mimi" (CJ's Grandmother and Aunt)** who gave me the most beautiful breast cancer centerpiece (a pink cup and saucer with a fashionably lady's high heel shoe). It sits in my living room today and reminds me of my fight. You too are a breast cancer survivor, and I thank you.

- **To Alice Harris** for preparing the most scrumptious healthy eating for us during my illness. We didn't realize that healthy foods could be so tasty.

- **To Doctors** Donald Block, Jennifer Amerson, Ira Robinson, Shyam Khanwani, Diane Alexander, Pamela Donlan, Russell Wilson, Kim Vu, Leticia Price, PA.; **GCS Nurses** Denise, Janise, Juan, Kim, Peggy, Felicia,

Melissa, Sherry, Carolyn and Zandra; **Radiation Oncology** Nurse Veda; **Plastic Surgeon** PA Pam & Nurse Merrell. You are all my heroes. Your phenomenal professionalism and kindness saved my life.

- **To Glenny Smith** for buying my very first wig. You made losing my hair less painful.
- **To Latoya Vinson, Sasha Vinson, Shelley Vinson Bullock**, together as "V-3". You sing like angels...YOU ROCK!
- **To Katie Shaw**, your gifts, visits and calls were priceless.
- **To Tammie Kincaid and Yolandia (Tish) Taylor.** You ladies were my endless reference guide taking me through every procedure, treatment, and surgery. Your own experiences with breast cancer were my pathway to get through this. Your stories are remarkable. You are true "survivors".
- **To Joyce Farmer.** You knew how much I loved Barbara Walters and "The View". Your gift to me of her book *"Audition"* was great reading while I was at home sick.

- **To Tim Owens.** As head of our Sound and Video team at my church, you made sure that I received a copy of dvds of the sermons and services that I missed while I was out sick. You don't know how much I love and appreciate you for it.
- **To Rose Saxon, Audrey Cohall, Deborah Ricks, Elder Vianna Harrison, Elder Joseph and Doris Whitaker, Adriana Moore, Barbara Deane-Redman, Bonita Houseworth, Christy Walker, Jennifer Duggan, Brenda Jackson, Vincent Smith, Shannon DeMyers, Simuel Flagg, Sona Chambers, Michele Ozumba, Vanessa Smalls, Kim Nolte, Andrea Sharpe, Don Mathis, Deverne Howell, Dr. Donna Elliston, Major Goggins, Debra Tucker, Jewell Jackson, Jennifer Driver, Tia Demery, Jim Stallard, Michael Benjamin, Adina Decouteau, Deidra Dukes, Ivy Styles, Justin Antoine, Francene Monenerkit, Monica Perez, Khatilia Harden, Shawna and Mike Brasfield, Elder Angela Mizell, Miriam Hester, Vickie Holmes, Trina Williams,** you

all were my life line via your many prayers, deeds, gifts, calls, and e-mails. Thank you for your love and care.

- **To my "Survivor Sisters":** Lucile Mosley (My Mom), Rosemary Hairston, Patricia (Patty) Fuchs, Germaine Lounds, Alicia Whitsett, Valerie Hawkins, Rhonda McKnight, Vanessa Blankenship along with the ones that have passed on; Tina Helms, Mrs. Johnson, Gwen James, Ruth Mackey ("Baby Sis"), Mother Bernice Murphy, Tracie McNabb and Aunt Vernell (Mosley) Bethel.

- **To Glenn (CJ) Baldwin and Herschel Symond.** You were my sons that helped my daughters get through the difficult times when I was sick.

- **To all my Caregroup Leader Sisters**, Liz Berry, Beverly Canady, Louvenia Willis, Lenette Day, Wilhelmina Hammond, Cheryl Goode, Pebbles Smith, Jesstine Evins, Kennitha Vaughn, Elder Tangela Allen, Lisa Harper, and Madelyn Hawwari. You are the most powerful prayer warriors ever.

SPECIAL DEDICATION

TO MY LOVING HUSBAND & CHILDREN

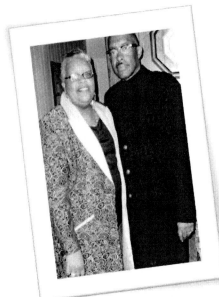

To my husband Paul, my daughters Dana and Brittanie, and four granddaughters: Zebria, Zoe, Amaya, and Jordynn. Paul, what can I say about your unconditional love. No one had to tell you what to do to love me, support me, be there for me to cry on your shoulder, or listen to my ramblings when I was so confused about my treatments. You only had to give me a look and I knew without discussion you supported my every decision. You never gave a second thought to accompany me to each doctors' visit I had to go to. You were there with me for every exam, procedure, treatment, and surgery...and you held my hand when I was SO afraid. I knew this was killing you inside, but not one time did you lose that warm embrace to assure me that everything would be alright... even when I learned later you cried often on other's shoulders. I thank you, and will never ever forget your sacrifice of love...just for me! To Janise, my stepdaughter. Your concern during my illness meant so much to me. I'll never forget the breast cancer replica trinkets you shared with me from your Pre-K students that brightened my days. To Dana, my oldest daughter. Your strength in prayer and

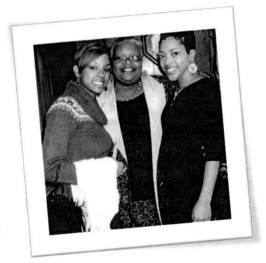

love was astronomical! You prayed like a warrior of true praise. I believe you and the

Lord had a bond of communication that not many have. You told me from the day I was diagnosed, that everything would be alright! You knew what I needed before I even asked...thank you for being there for me. To Brittanie, my baby girl. You were there sitting at my bedside when you came in from school or work and knew just the words to say to heal my heart. I'll never forget you going to the Cancer office with me that one visit and went into the treatment room with me to hold my hand through the drips...but instead snacked on all the treats for the patients and even went to sleep in one of the patients' treatment lounge chairs. The nurses thought you were so cute, and so did I. Thank you for going through this with me...you never left my side. To my, Zebria for telling me that I still looked cute with my bald head. To Zoe, when you learned I was writing my own book about my cancer experience, you decided that you'd write your own book as well. You were so fascinated on how the pages of a book came together. To Amaya, you too thought I looked pretty even without my hair. Your only concern, with that curious look on your face was...how am I going to now make "ponytails" with your hair since there is no more. Combing and playing in my hair was your favorite thing to do. And my little Jordynn. Your smile would light up the Brooklyn bridge. Your glow and little kisses on my face warmed my heart more than any love could. You grandgirls made my fight worth it all. I did it for you! I thank God for giving me such an incredible family!

RESOURCES

(Organizations that help Cancer Patients)

American Cancer Society

    www.cancer.org   1-800-227-2345

Cancer Care, Inc.

    www.cancercare.org   1-800-813-Hope

Cancer Hope Network

    www.cancerhopenetwork.org

                                       1-877-467-3638

Gilda's Club Worldwide

    www.gildasclub.org   1-888-445-3248

Sisters Network, Inc.
www.sistersnetworkinc.org
1-713-781-0255
(A National African-American Breast Cancer Survivor's Organization)

YWCA Encoreplus Program   www.ywca.org
1-800-953-7587

The Wellness Community
www.thewellnesscommunity.org

Y-ME National Breast Cancer Organization
www.y-me.org

1-800-221-2141 (English)*
1-800-986-9505 (Español)

SHARE: Self-Help for Women with Breast or Ovarian Cancer
www.sharecancersupport.org
1-212-382-2111 (English)

1-212-719-4454 (Spanish)

Faith in Action

www.fianationalnetwork.org

(Will run errands and assist at home)

Cleaning for a Reason

www.cleaningforareason.org

ABOUT THE AUTHOR

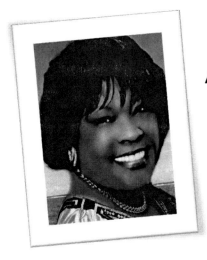

Althea Baldwin was born in Hallandale Beach, Florida. Her loving parents are Johnny Clarence, Sr. and Lucile Mosley. She is married to Paul Leon Baldwin and they are proud parents of three lovely and talented daughters and four beautiful granddaughters. Althea studied Business Administration and Accounting at Broward Jr. College and Georgia State University, which afforded her numerous opportunities in the Accounting field with corporations throughout the city of Atlanta, Georgia.

Althea is a member of Highpoint Christian Tabernacle Church in Smyrna, Georgia. As a devout member for over 20 years, Althea serves in various capacities including, the Women's Recording Choir, Pastors Aide and the Women's Caregroup Ministry, just to name a few. In her former church, Althea wrote several plays and skits and was faithfully active with women's groups.

Writing is enjoyable to Althea as she has written poetry, short stories, essays, and work-related job description manuals. Althea says writing is "like breathing fresh air". Therefore, when she was diagnosed with breast cancer, the composition of her very first book, **"The Day I No Longer 'Heard' The Sun Shine"** was birth!

In her own words… "This book is an opportunity to share with the world my personal testimony of the healing power of God…It is truly my desire that through my experience with breast cancer, I am able to minister to women on a deeper level about the faithfulness of God. It is my prayer that this book touches your life as much as it has touched mine."

CPSIA information can be obtained at www.ICGtesting.com
Printed in the USA
243802LV00002B/8/P